PLANT SPIRIT MEDICINE

PLANT SPIRIT
MEDICINE

Eliot Cowan

Swan•Raven & Company
An Imprint of Blue Water Publishing, Inc.
Box 726 Newberg, Oregon 97132
503/538-0264

Library of Congress Cataloging-in-Publication Data
Cowan, Eliot, 1946-
Plant Spirit Medicine / Eliot Cowan.

                          p. cm.

Includes bibliographical references.

                          I. Title.

F1221.H9C69 1995
615.8'8' 0972--dc20   95-5643
                                                        CIP

ISBN 0-926524-09-7 : $13.95
                        1. Huichol Indians--Ethnobotany.
                        2. Huichol Indians--Medicine.
                        3. Huichol Indians--Religion.
                        4. Ethnobotany--Mexico.
                        5. Medicinal plants--Mexico.
                        6. Healing--Mexico.
                        7. Shamanism--Mexico.

Design Implementation: Carlene Lynch
Book Design: Marcia Barrentine
Book Cover Design: Pamela Meyer and Brian L. Crissey
Biographical Photo: Dennis Davis
Back Cover Photo: Jonathan Finegold

Printed in the United States of America
Address all inquiries   Swan•Raven & Co.
                                         P. O. Box 726
                                         Newberg, OR 97132
                                         U.S.A.

Swan•Raven & Co. has made the commitment to use 100% recycled paper whenever possible.

Acknowledgments

My wife Victoria and our children Briana, Aura, Omar, and Victoria Liliana went many days without husband or father to make this book possible. For their tolerant, magnanimous hearts I offer deepest gratitude.

Professor J. R. Worsley, Carolyn Carr, Michael Harner, Don José Ríos, Don José Morales, Don Guadalupe González, Muktananda Swami, and Chidvilasananda Swami all helped show the way. May everyone find such magnificent teachers!

My patients and students inspired me with their faith and pioneer spirit. These wonderful people are too many to thank by name, but I would single out Robin Bisio, the first person to receive plant spirit medicine through me.

My brother Ish gave safe harbor to my soul, believed in me, and always had the right words to say. He is father and mother to this book and to many other things I have done.

A number of friends and colleagues offered home, food, labor or transportation to help bring plant spirit medicine out of the closet. My admiration and thanks go to John Pope, Victoria Goldbach and Dennis Davis, Ron Puhky, Sharon Puhky-Evans, Donna Guillemin, Joyce Netishen, Dr. Gil Milner, Casey Carter, Suzanne Burnell, Susan Reed, Megan Godfrey, Pat Gorman, the late Professor Patrick Watson, Fabienne Alsing and Professor J. R. Worsley.

The enthusiasm of Gary Hardin, Gerhard Riemann and Rachel Farber saved the manuscript from oblivion. Ms. Farber's keen mind and gentle ways made her the ideal editor. David Kyle of Swan•Raven & Co. offered the book not just a house, but a home.

On behalf of everyone who receives their help, I offer astonished thanks to the plant spirits who come through my hands.

Finally, my love and gratitude go to the One who answers my prayers even before I know how to utter them.

Author's Prefatory Note

I thought about this book for almost a year before I actually sat down to it. The day I began writing was the day I was told I would be introduced to Don Guadalupe González Ríos, a Huichol Indian shaman. Somehow this news gave me energy. There was a sensation of having the wind at my back, speeding me somewhere I wanted very much to go.

As it turns out, that sensation was quite accurate. Among the Huichols, "wind" is the symbol for the unseen and all-pervasive power of a shaman, and Don Guadalupe received his gifts from a plant so holy that his people call it the "wind tree."

Perhaps years of work prepared me to meet this man. When he began to teach me about the blessings of the wind tree, I was ready to hear his message. I had seen it over and over again: gracious plant spirits liberating people from suffering. Or perhaps I was prepared to meet him by the very suffering of people who don't know where to look for grace.

Don Guadalupe's plant teachers filled his heart with a love that illness can not withstand, a love that make him an unshakable, happy man. He wants to share that love with me, and with you, if you care to have it. It comes in compassionately measured doses during several years of muscle-building apprenticeship.

If the story of my apprenticeship is to be told, it will have to wait. In the meantime, this book comes to you on the breeze of the wind tree. It is a personal book full of stories, but it is only incidentally about my colleagues and me. The book is really about how the Creator's love medicine flows to you through our brothers and sisters who have roots. If my prayers have been answered, the book is that love and that medicine.

Table Of Contents

Foreward

by Hal Zina Bennett, Ph.D.

Hal Zina Bennett is the author and/or co-author of more than 30 success-ful books on holistic health, spirituality and human consciousness. His most recent books are Zuni Fetishes: Using Native American Objects for Med-itation, Reflection and Insight, *and* Lens of Perception, *a breakthrough book on human consciousness and the powers of perception.*

I first met Eliot Cowan nearly ten years ago, when I was asked to work with him on an article on plant spirit medicine for Shaman's Drum magazine. At the time, he had been working with plant spirits for less than three years. He'd been getting excellent results from his ef-forts and was attempting to integrate what he was learning with his very successful work as an acupuncturist in Sacramento.

I was intrigued by Eliot's writings, in part because of my own in-terest in holistic health and shamanism. I had read about the healings of indigenous peoples throughout the world who cured with plant spirits, and the process had intrigued me. However, the idea that plants have spirits and that humans are capable of communicating with them ran against the grain of all I'd been taught through my formal educa-tion. Yet, it was clear from talking and reading about healings that had taken place in this way, that there was something to it and that people truly had received miraculous healings through the medicine men and women who practiced this process.

There is a part of me that even now holds onto my faith in the sci-entific method, insisting on *proof*, at least in the form of well document-ed empirical evidence. Yet, my own experiences with ancient shamanistic practices long ago convinced me that there is an unseen re-ality which impacts our lives profoundly, yet which science has been unable to validate. The work I did with Eliot Cowan on his first article opened my eyes and I began looking at plants in a new way. I had al-ways felt nurtured in nature, feeling the spirit of the forests during walks in the woods, and recognizing how very deeply touched I was by flowers or by eating vegetables freshly picked from our own garden. Perhaps, I reasoned, my responses to the vegetable world went deeper than aesthetics.

While I did not see or speak with the spirits of plants—at least not in the way Eliot describes in this book—I definitely began to change how I related to plants. Clearly, they were *animate*; that is, they contained and expressed the spirit of life which lives in all of us and which is the essence of the mystery of life itself. And clearly, each plant appeared to project an identify of its own—a character, if you will, that told what it was about. When I began looking very closely, I became convinced that the character of each plant was something much more than an aesthetic judgment on my part. I found myself deeply attracted, for example, to stinging nettle which grew in abundance along a walking trail I discovered during a camping trip in Northern California. It was clearly not a beautiful plant, with its rather forbidding, spiked leaves that left your skin burning if you brushed against them. However, I somehow knew this plant had a generous and helpful spirit. During one wilderness trip, we were plagued by mosquitoes and when I looked around for a way to relieve the itching welts that covered my body, I found myself focusing in on the nettle growing along a little creek. I carefully picked a couple dozen leaves, put them into a pot, covered them with water, and steamed them for about twenty minutes. Then I swabbed my skin with the still warm, damp leaves, which by now looked a little like overcooked spinach. Almost instantly the itching stopped and the mosquito welts went down. My partner did the same and also enjoyed relief.

Later, back at the trailhead, I spoke with other campers about our experience with the nettle. An older couple said that they, too, used the "stinging nettle" for this purpose. In addition, they told us that a tea made from the nettle was an excellent remedy for diarrhea and that it was reputed to be excellent for stimulating the immune system to help deal with infection. Another woman told us that the cooked leaves of nettle are quite tasty and that she always mixed them with the dried backpacking foods she carried with her into the mountains.

As I became increasingly aware of the complexity of our relationships with the plant world, I began to ask a brand new set of questions. First and foremost, I had growing respect for the ancient tradition of herbology for healing, which was actually the basis for modern pharmaceuticals—and continues to have a major impact on that field. I asked myself, how did the first ancient healers learn of the medicinal benefits of foxglove, for example, that was later the basis for formulating *digitalis*, for treating certain heart disease? Unlikely that it was discovered randomly, through accident or trial and error. It seemed reasonable to assume that ancient medicine men or women were somehow able to communicate with the plants or in some other intuitive way *read* what they might offer us humans.

I continued to be interested in how we humans discovered the benefits of plants. Then, toward the end of my mother's life, she mentioned to me that her grandmother, who lived in Northern Michigan, had been a midwife and herbalist. I had never heard this story before. I asked my mother if she knew how my great grandmother learned about such things. Had she studied with another healer? Mother didn't know the answer to that, but she said that the her grandmother often went foraging in the woods and meadows for her herbs and that she seemed to have a reverence for the plants, treating them as if they were god-given, almost like angels sent to help humans. She said that her grandmother also told her that animals are able to communicate with plants, that a dog or cat, for example, will seek out exactly the right plants and eat them for their therapeutic effects. Mother said that when her own mother hemorrhaged following childbirth, her grandmother gathered herbs near their home and administered them, stopping the bleeding almost immediately.

Upon first reading the manuscript for this book, I was reminded of all these events, most of which I'd experienced or had been told about since my first work with Eliot several years before. Now I saw that he had taken his research a giant step further. He had gone off to study with healers such as Don José Ríos, Don José Morales, and Don Guadalupe González and others, and he had come back with information that has been lost to the modern world. Moreover, there were new elements to his work—the use of shamanic dreams to help guide and direct the therapeutic process using plants. All of this indicated to me that unlike so many modern whites who have become intrigued by shamanism and the ways of indigenous peoples, Eliot had gone the full route. He had done his homework in a sober and thorough way, seeking answers not because he was drawn by some sentimental notion about "Indian ways," or the ways of ancient intuitive societies but because he was genuinely interested in healing. He seemed driven by a mission to do the very best he could to find the most effective use of healing plants.

I read this manuscript from front to back, pulled along, page after page, by the author's modesty, thoroughness and dedication to his subject. Halfway through, I realized that this man was probably the most "authentic" student of the ancient ways that I had ever read. He not only didn't sensationalize or sentimentalize his teachers, he unflinch-

xvi 🦋 *Plant Spirit Medicine*

ingly observed their shortcomings when they were displayed, gleaning their wisdom in spite of themselves. He confronted his own skepticism and moved beyond it to discover and ultimately begin practicing and teaching to others all that he had learned.

I believe we all owe Eliot a great debt of gratitude. Many people have spoken of the importance of going into the remote areas of the world where herbal healing and shamanism are still alive and well, though quickly dying out as a result of civilization encroaching upon their habitats. Drug companies are spending millions of dollars going into the diminishing rain forests, seeking chemical compounds of the healing plants. Yet, here is Eliot, a single man, who has not only studied very hard with the ancient healers but himself has become a gifted healer and teacher, sharing his valuable gifts with all of us.

This is a breakthrough book in its own right, filled with stories of the adventures of this healer, but also filled with wisdom that might have been lost forever had it not been for Eliot's courage, burning curiosity and desire to be of real service, that motivated him to dedicate his life to this craft. Eliot is a modern man who has found a way to seek out the wisdom of the past and bring it into a contemporary setting before it is lost forever. His work restores our link with the powers of ancient intuitive traditions which can serve us in our lives today. And his efforts add to our collection of tools for mending not only our individual health complaints but also the violent wound that has severed us from the natural world and the world of spirit.

Part 1

Plants, Spirits
and Their Medicine

Plant Spirit Medicine Dreams

My friend Peter Gorman is walking down a trail in the Amazon jungle. He is on his way back to the village after watching his Matses Indian friend set a trap for wild boar. The Indian takes advantage of the walk to show Peter some medicinal plants growing along the trail. Within a few minutes he has pointed out several dozen species and pantomimed their healing virtues.

Arriving at the village, Peter summons his interpreter and returns to the hunter's hut. He didn't have his notebook with him on the walk, he explains, and he couldn't possibly remember all he had been shown. Would the hunter be kind enough to say once again how the herbs were prepared and used?

The hunter-shaman smiles at Peter and then begins to laugh. He invites all his wives and children over to have a good laugh, too. When they have all laughed themselves out, he explains, "That was just to introduce you to some of the plants. If you want to actually use a plant yourself, the spirit of the plant must come to you in your dreams. If the spirit of the plant tells you how to prepare it and what it will cure, you can use it. Otherwise, it won't work for you. Boy, that was a good one! I've got to remember what you just said!" He laughs again.

Meanwhile, in Connecticut, a major pharmaceutical firm approaches a shamanic studies institute. The firm wants to contact shamans of the Amazon in order to get information on medicinal plants. The company plans to take samples of the herbs, isolate active molecules, and manufacture them in the laboratory.

I can imagine the scene when the pharmaceutical firm makes it to the Amazon: The shamans laughing uproariously as they collect their fees. The field workers rushing specimens back to the laboratory. Skilled technicians spending millions of company dollars researching new compounds, only to come up with one disappointment after another. The shamans will be discredited, but they won't care. They will still be in the jungle working cures with the plants they have used for centuries.

The American firm will go to the jungle infatuated with its superior technology, dreaming of profits from a patentable new drug. No one will think of asking the shamans what the active ingredients are. If they do ask, they won't like the answer.

There is only one active ingredient in plant medicines—friendship. A plant spirit heals a patient as a favor to its friend-in-dreaming, the doctor.

To the people of the Amazon this truth is basic. Any four-year-old understands it. That is why the Matses hunter-shaman called his children over to have a good laugh at my friend Peter. They couldn't believe a grown man could be so silly!

The Matses and many other non-European peoples understand that both nature and humankind are endowed with intelligence and spirit. Therefore, humans and nature are of the same family. In all cultures there exist individuals who have especially vivid experiences with the spirits of nature. These are the shamans. Shamans make friends of the spirits of nature and call upon them for help with everyday affairs.

Plant spirit medicine is the shaman's way with plants. It recognizes that plants have spirit, and that spirit is the strongest medicine. Spirit can heal the deepest reaches of the heart and soul.

There is nothing exotic about all this. Don't be misled by talk about the Amazon. If you want to meet the most powerful healing plants in the world, just open your door and step outside. They are growing all around you. If you don't believe me, or if you have a taste for romantic locations, you can try going elsewhere. But if you stay there long enough, it comes down to the same thing: dealing with the local weeds.

In keeping with this homegrown quality, I want to tell you what has been happening around my home lately. At first this may seem to have nothing to do with our subject, but bear with me; in time it will make sense.

Today I went to visit a Huichol Indian named José Benítez Sánchez. In certain circles José is famous as a visionary artist. Among his own people he is known as a shaman. José lives part-time in a village near Tepic, Mexico. The rest of the time he lives in the resort city of Puerto Vallarta. It was there I went to find him.

As I approached his home in one of the humblest districts in town, I recalled the first time I met José the year before. This was a man who earned a huge income by Indian standards. Yet as he welcomed me into his house, it was apparent that he had but one material possession of any consequence—an electric fan. Our visit was brief, for he was due to leave in a few hours to meet with the President of Mexico.

José cheerfully admitted that he did not have money for bus fare. Looking down at his ragged cut-offs, he allowed that he also did not own a pair of pants to wear to greet the President. Evidently he sensed I was confused about why a successful man should be so destitute, for he told me the following story:

> When I was a boy I admired my grandfather. He was a powerful shaman. One day when he felt I was old enough to understand, he told me, "José, there are two types of power that one can acquire. One type is used for your own personal reasons. The other is used for the benefit of your people. You can walk the road to the first type of power or the second. But let me tell you this: the second road is the road to happiness." Since my grandfather was a very wise man, I took his advice, and I have stayed on the second road. Whenever the gods give me something, I immediately pass it on for the use of my people.

José's presence radiated contentment. Obviously his grandfather had known what he was talking about. I dug into my suitcase and came up with a pair of pants, which I presented to him together with his bus fare. He accepted my gifts with sincere thanks and not a trace of surprise. Then he took off on his voyage to see the President, leaving me one small step farther down the road to happiness.

As I was reminiscing about that first meeting, I looked up to see José walking toward me. José is a good-looking, compact man of middle years. Today he was wearing long pants, a short-sleeved shirt and a cowboy hat. The only sign of his background was his intensely colorful Huichol shoulder bag.

He invited me into his house. We sat down at a table with two of his paintings-in-progress. We chatted about the pilgrimage he would be leading in a few days. Children toddled in and out. A teenage girl stood outside, her chin propped on the windowsill, listening carefully. Eventually I got around to the purpose of my visit:

"I want to ask your advice about something, Don José."

"Of course. Go ahead."

"Did you know an old man, a great shaman named Don José Ríos? They called him Matsuwa."

"Matsuwa, yes. He was a relative of mine."

"Well, I met him years ago, and he helped me. Then, about three years ago, my father was dying of cancer. He said he wanted a shaman to help him, so I went to see Matsuwa. He was living in Las Blancas at that time."

José nodded.

"When I arrived I found that Matsuwa was as bad off as my father was. He was very weak and couldn't get out of bed. He was moaning with pain; he said that his legs were killing him. He was lying in the hot sun, but he was shivering with cold. I had to put a blanket over him."

José made a face to let me know he understood the anguish of the moment.

"It occurred to me to see if I could help Matsuwa. I gave him a treatment. Right away he stopped shivering and asked to have the blanket taken off. His legs stopped hurting too, although he was still too weak to sit up. When the people saw this they asked me if I could help them too. One of Matsuwa's nephews took me to see his father, who had been hit by a train and couldn't walk. On the way to see his father, the boy asked me if I believed in the Huichol way of healing, using feathers. I said, yes, of course I believed in it. 'In fact,' I told him, 'your uncle helped me a lot with his feathers. I would like to learn about Huichol healing myself.'

"The boy told me that there was someone in the village who was very good at healing with feathers. This man had learned his skill by making a pilgrimage every year for five years to a nearby peak."

"That peak is called 'El Picacho,'" said José.

"You know it, then," I said.

"Of course."

"Well, after that I returned to the United States, and I began to visit El Picacho in my dreams. I want to tell you what I saw in my dreams, so that you can advise me, Don José."

"What did you see?" José asked me.

"At the very top of the mountain there is a flat area where two trees grow. There is a person there, a Huichol man. He is short. His face is round; he has plump cheeks. He smiles all the time. The little man is accompanied by a small deer. The deer dances and does all sorts of antics. The deer and the man let me know that they can help me to heal people.

"I have dreamed of this place many times now. There have been occasions when people who live far away have asked me to heal them. Since I didn't know what else to do, I have asked the man and the deer to do the work. There have been some very good results."

"It is exactly as you say," said José.

"What do you mean?" I asked.

"The tree you saw is the wind tree that grows on that peak. The short man lives there too. He is the magic of the wind tree. If you go there he will talk to you, just as we are talking. But you should tell him to talk with you in Spanish, because you don't understand Huichol.

"I have seen this little Huichol man. He crosses my path when I am on pilgrimage to visit the gods. I ask his permission to pass. I explain that I am on my way to someplace else, and he lets me go. Just as you say, he is very short and has fat cheeks and thick lips. Actually he is very, very old, although often he appears to be young. The deer lives there at El Picacho as well. Sometimes the antlers of the deer appear on the head of the little man. This is all the magic of the wind tree, which you also saw in your dream. The wind tree teaches people how to heal. It also teaches music. There is a world-famous musician in our tribe. It was the wind tree that taught him."

"You say that a wind tree grows on the peak," I said, "but there were two trees in my vision."

"They are both the wind tree," José replied. "One represents the left antlers of the deer and the other represents the right antlers. Many people go and make the sacrifice to the wind tree there at El Picacho. This is a very good thing. Because you have dreamed this, it would be very good for you to go. The little man you saw does live there. If you go with faith and ask that he appear to you so that you can learn from him, he will appear in person.

"However, it would be necessary to consult first with someone who is familiar with the magic of El Picacho, someone who has made the sacrifice. I myself rarely go to that region. I keep busy with other sacrifices, other pilgrimages. There is someone in my village, though, who knows the mountain very well. His name is Guadalupe González Ríos, and he is also related to José Ríos. He is a very good man, not at all stingy with information. I am going to our village tomorrow. When I see him, immediately I will remember this conversation and I will tell him about you. Perhaps you can come to the fiesta when we return from our pilgrimage. The three of us can talk together then. We should be back by the 24th."

"What day of the week is that?"

"Thursday, I believe."

"Friday!" said the girl in the window. This was her first contribution to the conversation.

"Too bad!" I said. "I will be in the United States at that time."

"Never mind. Come by my house when you return and we will go to my village together. Perhaps I will bring along another man who has also dreamed of the wind tree. He is a German."

"Frenchman," chimed the girl.

More than once during my school years, I awoke in the middle of the night with the solution to a mathematical equation that had completely stumped me during the day. I never told anyone that I had done my algebra homework in my sleep. I was afraid that people would think I was weird. Eventually I stopped having these dreams.

Much later in life I discovered that it is not at all unusual for people to learn from dreams. Nowadays I enjoy asking people if they have ever dreamed something which later came to pass. About seventy-five percent say they have indeed had a dream of this type. And everyone has dreams that take place somewhere other than the bedroom where their sleeping body lies. When we dream we can easily travel to distant places. We can know the future. We are given special understanding that enables us to solve life's problems.

For the most part these wonderful dream powers lie "dormant" in our society, but the Huichols and the Matses of the Amazon consider dream learning to be "true" learning. Indeed nearly every culture on earth, except our own, respects dream learning as true learning. We revere the rational, analytical method of learning honed and polished since the days of the ancient Greeks. We do not realize that the shamans of our species have honed and polished another method. This dreaming method is neither rational nor analytical, but it works extremely well.

The key to this method is to get into the dream state of consciousness, keeping in mind what it is that you wish to learn or accomplish. The way you get into the dream state is incidental. Some shamans learn to go to sleep and dream about what they wish to dream about. Others use psychotropic plants. Many simply listen to monotonous drumming to induce the dream state. I use drumming.

When I first heard about El Picacho several years ago, I was eager to learn from the spirits said to dwell there. With the demands of conducting a busy acupuncture practice, raising young children, and attending my dying father, it was impossible to visit the peak in person, so I decided to visit in dreams. I lit a candle and some incense to help set the mood, then I lay down on my back and relaxed. I affirmed my intention to visit the sacred site and meet any helpful spirits that might live there. As I listened to loud, repetitive drumbeats, my state of consciousness shifted. My dream helpers appeared to me and flew me to the peak where I had the experiences I recounted to José Benítez Sánchez today, several years after the original dream.

My conversation with José confirmed for me that my dream corresponds with an ancient tradition. As a Huichol and a shaman, he had no trouble accepting that I had met a tree spirit who could help me heal people. Being a middle-class white American, on the other hand, I have been plagued for years with the question: "Am I making this up?"

"Am I making this up?" This is the question, the monster, faced by every Westerner who ventures into the world of dreams. There is only one way to subdue this monster—put the dream to the test and see if it works. If the magic of the wind tree can heal people, does it really matter whether I am making it up?

Several years ago, I guided a group of my students to dream the medicine of the willow. We were sitting in a circle sharing our dreams. One man, a physician, said that there was an aspect of his dream he did not know how to interpret. "Over and over again," he said, "the willow spirit kept repeating to me, 'Look up! Look up! Always look up!'"

A month later I again met with the physician, who told the following story:

> I have a patient who seemed perfect for willow medicine, so I've given it to her three times now. When she came back after the first treatment, she insisted I tell her what that "wonderful medicine" was. At the same time she kept turning to a potted willow on my windowsill. She said something strange and wonderful: "That plant is so lovely. I would like to be that plant!"
>
> I asked her to tell me what the treatment had done for her, and she mentioned improvements in a long list of physical complaints. "But," she said, "This is the best thing of all…. I didn't realize it before, but I have been depressed all my life. I was so negative! It was as if my mind's eye was always looking down at the ground, and all I could see was the dirt. But you know, from the moment I left here last time, I heard a voice inside that said, 'Look up! Look up! Always look up!' and now it's as if I am seeing the beauty around me for the first time!"
>
> At that moment I told her that the plant on the windowsill and the medicine she had taken were both willow. I also shared with her my willow dream and said I had heard the same voice saying, "Look up!" She was so moved she began to cry. At the next treatment she

brought in a poem she had written to thank the willow spirit.

The experiences of the class, the physician, the patient—where did they come from? Is there such a thing as a willow spirit? If so, what is it really? Does it matter? Evidently it *does* matter to the young physician. He has since decided that we were all just making it up, and he has stopped practicing plant spirit medicine.

As for me, it seems that plant spirit medicine keeps practicing me. I thought I would go to José Benítez Sánchez and find out about an entirely different kind of healing having to do with sacred mountains, dancing deer, and such. I instead found out it is all about the magic of the wind tree, so I'm back where I started from—learning medicine from plants.

Plants

The year is 1970. I am an urban expatriate trying to live on the land in Northern Vermont. It is early spring; there is still snow on the ground. Soon it will be time to fix the fence, and I need posts. I shoulder a bow saw and a machete and set off to my favorite part of the farm—the cedar bog that surrounds the waterfall.

The sun is shining brightly today, although the air is still cool. As I enter the woods I listen to the wind sifting through the cedar boughs. I take a pinch of leaves, crush them under my nose, and nod a greeting to the trees. The cedars here grow in little families with several trunks sharing their roots. Among these families are miniature meadows, soon to be filled with grasses and wildflowers. I will spend the next two or three days working in this place, I guess. Had I brought the chain saw, I could have been finished by lunchtime today. Dinner at the latest. I make a mental note never to bring the chain saw.

I have never cut fence posts by myself before. This time I can do it any way I want. How do I want to do it? If I were growing here in this bog, how would I want it done? I turn to the nearest cedar and ask it how I should cut the fence posts. I don't expect an answer, of course, and I don't get one. Or do I? Somehow it is now perfectly obvious how I will cut my posts. From each clump I will select a trunk that is crowding the others. I will carefully cut that trunk, limb it, and pile the brush on top of the stump. This way, I won't kill a single tree, I won't choke the meadows with brush piles, and I will leave the grove healthier and more beautiful than I found it. This will probably take me an extra day or so, but who cares?

Poet Gary Snyder says the way we kill our farm animals is a source of endless bad luck for our society. This is an interesting statement and, I think, a true one. It is based on an understanding of what in the East is called the law of karma. Here in the West, we express the same understanding through homilies: "What goes around, comes around." "He who lives by the sword shall die by the sword." Many people have expressed concern and even outrage at the unnatural and cruel lives and deaths inflicted upon our livestock. It took Snyder, who is no vegetarian, to point out that our behavior towards animals rebounds on us just like all the rest of our behavior. If we take lives without respect and gratitude for the sacrificed animals, then we too will be subject to humiliation and alienation. This is not cruel fate or harsh nature, but just us creating our own bad luck.

Might it not be also worthwhile to consider our relationship to plants? The most striking thing about this relationship is that we need them but they don't need us. We humans are utterly dependent on plants to cover all our needs: fuel, shelter, clothing, medicine, the petrochemical cornucopia, and, of course, food. (Even meat is made of plants.) In contrast, plant communities do just fine without people. We seem to offer plants nothing but suffering, destruction and the threat of extinction.

There is some karmic rebound here. We are devastating forests and the foundations of vegetable life: soil, air, water and solar radiation. This is not only murderous, but also suicidal. Under the circumstances, the continued generosity of plants towards our species is absolutely remarkable. What makes plants so generous? What makes us so brutal?

Somewhere along the way we lost the experience of unity. We live our lives propping up the pathetic lie that we are different from everything else. This is a lie because the same awareness shines in the heart of all things. The lie is pathetic because it dooms us to a dry life of alienation.

Difference breeds indifference. If you think the forest is not you, you are more willing to exploit it or let others exploit it for you.

Plants, on the other hand, are not under the illusion that they are separate from the rest of creation. Observe how any plant interacts with soil, air, minerals, animals and insects. Everything around it is enriched and benefited by its presence. Plants live in harmony with nature. One might even say that plants are nature. Out of this union comes their incredible generosity to us and to all their other fellow creatures.

For the first time I am dreaming with a plant. English plantain is growing here, and I see a young woman with enormous wings sprouting from her shoulders. Somehow I know she is the plantain spirit. I approach her and introduce myself. She asks why I have come.

"First of all, " I reply, "I want to thank you for the help you have given my friends and me over the years. Your leaves have healed many wounds. I come to visit you to ask for another kind of help, a deeper kind. The cuts and

scrapes of my people are nothing compared to the pain in our hearts and the pollution in our minds. Can you help relieve this kind of suffering too?"

The plantain woman hops off her leaf and flies close to me. For a moment she hovers in front of my face and looks intently into my eyes. Then she smiles and says, "Of course, I will help you. My brothers and sisters will help you also. We are very happy to do this. In fact, we have been waiting for two hundred years for someone to ask us for this kind of help. We can do nothing unless we are asked."

"We can do nothing unless we are asked." Leave it to a plant to come up with the understatement of the millennium! Look at what plants do when they are asked: all human civilization is a form of excess grain—the generosity of plants. The history of our species shows us that plants furnish us with whatever we ask for. Our society values comfort, so that is what we have gone to the plant world to get. This is wonderful as far as it goes, which is not very far in the direction of satisfaction. If for a moment we could forget the quest for comfort and ask plants to help us find joy, richness and significance in life, is there any reason to suppose they would not share those qualities with us just as they have shared everything else? To think that plants are mere dumb creatures that do not know ecstasy is ignorance or tragic arrogant folly.

All things enjoy ecstatic union with nature. Life without ecstasy is not true life and not worth living. Without ecstasy the soul becomes shriveled and perverted, the mind becomes corrupt and the body suffers pain. Ecstatic union with nature is necessary for normal health. It is necessary for survival.

I gave a class recently in which the students brought patients for me to treat. One of the patients was a middle-aged man just out of the hospital. He suffered from leukemia and had had a close brush with death. He had abandoned his artistic career and was wandering about looking for a treatment that could spare him pain in his last days. A dream journey to his soul revealed an inner landscape barren and forlorn as the most forbidding desert. I treated this man with the spirits of two plants. A few days later, I returned home to Mexico. Before long, I got this letter from the student who followed up on his treatment:

> The man we saw earlier this month who had leukemia called me this week saying he had felt good results from the treatment and wanted to come see me for another treatment. When he came, he began to tell me what had happened to him. The day following your treatment with him he awoke in what he called "a differ-

ent state of consciousness," which has been constantly with him ever since. He spoke of "recollecting himself" by going to an island where his family had spent a lot of time, and also to a petroglyph that was an important rock to him and had at one time spoken to him.

Last week his doctor reduced his white cell killing drug by one half because his white cell count had dropped by one half. He cleaned up his studio and has begun painting again. He has been having what he calls "lucid dreams," and he speaks of the healing quality of these dreams.

Anticipating his treatment, I had decided to use the mullein spirit with him. The day before he arrived I had found mullein growing in a ravine. The following morning before he got to my house, I made another dream journey to the mullein. I was transported to a place where a crow waited for me alongside a colony of mullein plants. Nearby, a tree was standing. Among its limbs, crow feathers and mullein leaves formed a nest. Here someone needing nurturing would be fulfilled with waves of blessings. When he was ready he would then fly away.

When our patient arrived I treated him with the mullein spirit. As he was lying on the table he heard a crow outside my window. He began telling a story of having taken a baby crow that was once given to a girlfriend of his. She not wanting it, our patient made a nest for it and cared for it for months. He spoke of how deeply he became involved, learning the ways of crows. When the time came, the crow flew away.

The most remarkable thing in this story is that the patient entered a "different state of consciousness." This new consciousness enabled him to find healing in his dreams. It enabled him to re-enter the magical connection with nature that he had had in his youth. Inside that magic, life was once again worth living, and his body responded by rallying to fight his disease. The proof that this man was healed was that he cleaned up his studio and began to paint once again. In other words, he was resurrected. He came back to life.

Thanks to ecstatic union with nature, this man now has some chance of survival, whereas before, he had none. Ultimately, though, healing is not about whether you die. Healing is about how fully you live. I hope this artist goes on to live a long and fruitful life, but if he were to die tomorrow, he would still be a great success because he would have really lived.

For my protection and your enlightenment, it is worth taking a moment to make sure this is clear: I did *not* diagnose or treat this man for leukemia. Plant spirit medicine does not diagnose or treat any illness. I am not holding out any herbal preparation as a cure for any disease. In chapter twelve I will further explain how the practitioner of plant spirit medicine, in assessing which plants to use with a given person, pays no attention whatsoever to any symptoms that person may have.

There are many examples of plants' willingness to reintroduce us to the joy of a close relationship with nature. A sixteen-year-old boy, for example, came to see me complaining of severe hay fever. Since he worked part-time as a gardener, this was a serious handicap. After his first treatment he returned and asked me what was that "weird stuff" I had given him. I asked him why he thought it was weird, and he replied that on his way home from my office all the trees and shrubs "were, like, waving at me and stuff!" I knew immediately that the plants were signaling their friendliness to him and that their pollen would no longer cause him any trouble. This turned out to be true.

Other people have returned after treatment to tell me stories of "falling in love with the Earth," or "feeling like I'm not alone," or "seeing fairies in my backyard." One of my favorite such stories involves Karen, a woman in her twenties who was suffering from depression as well as a number of physical complaints. I had chosen to treat her with the spirit of hummingbird sage, a beautiful shrub that grows in the coastal ranges of Southern California, where I was living at the time. In my dream work with the hummingbird sage, the spirit appeared to me as a jolly, muscular little man full of fun and kindness. He was dressed in a pointed cap, a medieval tunic, leggings and shoes with pointy turned-up toes.

This was Karen's report after her treatment:

> After I left here I felt so tired that I went home and lay down. I was half asleep and had a dream or a daydream or something. It was totally vivid and lifelike. In this dream I felt that someone else was entering my body. I wasn't frightened because I felt he was a very good person—kind and fun-loving. I could see him very clearly. He was short and strong and was wearing funny old-

fashioned clothing and shoes with pointy, turned-up toes. I felt he was there to give me something I needed.

That afternoon I felt a strong urge to go to my special spot in the mountains. There is a certain place I go to; the smell there reminds me of the smell of the sage that grows in Colorado, in the Rockies. I lived in Colorado until my mother died. I don't know, I guess I am trying to recapture the feeling about life that I used to have when my mother was alive, so I go to this place. The problem is, I never quite manage to get the feeling back. I get a little glimpse of it, but then it fades away. But this time, after the treatment I went to my spot and it worked! I got that wonderful feeling back! In fact it still hasn't left me!

I asked Karen to draw me a detailed map of her special spot in the mountains. After work I drove up there and hiked to the exact location. There I found one of the largest stands I'd ever seen of the fragrant hummingbird sage.

Some people, like Karen, are sensitive to these experiences and communicate them well. Others are less sensitive, less articulate. Many people probably never tell me about them because they don't want me to think they are crazy. Nevertheless, I have heard many of these stories, and I now believe that everyone who is touched by the plant spirits gets some taste of magic and union with nature. The following excerpt is from a letter written by another observant and expressive woman. She writes of the effects of her first treatment:

...It was wonderful—no, better than that, it was fantastic, magical, incredible and, to top it all, you (or rather the spirits) cured me of a deep and dark longing that I have carried with me like a pain all my life. I feel that something has become clearer, has settled, is no longer a question, a separation. Since I last saw you, many strange and magical things have happened to me—dreams and unusual coincidences. All of it confirms for me what I have always believed—that everything is connected, all are part of the whole. I have always known this but did not directly experience it. But since your treatment it is as if many doors have been pulled open and the spirit allowed to rush in. I feel "touched," connected, whole, and a little mad—intoxicated, full of joy!

Plants wish us well in every way. They can provide not only for our physical needs, but also for our heart and soul. They are perfectly willing to bring us into the blessings of their union with nature. But, as the plantain spirit told me, they can do nothing unless they are asked. I would add that we have to know the right questions and the right way to ask them.

What is the right way to ask a plant? Part of it has to do with appreciating that a plant has roots. A plant lives here, with this dirt, rain, sunshine and air. With these it does its growth magic. From plants we learn that if you want to enter nature, you have to do it here because this is the only place nature can be found. From this it follows that if you are going to ask a plant to bring you into the blessing of nature, you have to ask a plant that grows here. J. R. Worsley, the great English acupuncturist, says, "Local herbs are not ten times stronger, not a hundred times stronger. Local herbs are *one thousand times* stronger than exotic ones!" Professor Worsley is not exaggerating.

One woman described her first treatment with (local) plant spirit medicine as "bringing me back to a place I've been before." This gets right to the crux. We are part of nature, but how many of us really live in nature? Whether we live in mud huts or skyscrapers is not entirely the point. The point is the joy of being in the dance of creation as an equal partner with everything. This means bringing us back to where we already live—on the earth, with the dirt, the rain, the sunshine and the air, just like our brothers and sisters, the plants.

After her first plant spirit medicine treatment, one of my patients said she felt that for two weeks she was on the verge of receiving some sort of a "spiritual message." At the second session I gave her mountain mahogany. The spirit of this plant appears to me as a wise old Native American Grandmother. She comes from a tribe that performs ceremonies in underground chambers. I was hoping this Grandmother would be able to give my patient the instruction she needed, for Grandmothers are guardians and teachers of traditional spiritual lore.

After the mountain mahogany treatment, Glenda, my patient, started hearing two words repeating constantly in her head. She had never heard them together and had no idea what they meant: "Second Mesa."

The following day she was watching television with her husband. It was a documentary on the Hopi Indians, and they both found it very interesting. After it was over she turned to him and said, "That's it! The Hopis! Someone there has the message for me! Darling, we've got to go visit the Hopis!"

"Fine, dear, that's wonderful! But where will we go? I don't know where the Hopis live, do you?"

"How am I supposed to know? You know I've never been out of California in my life!"

"Well, I'll go get the road atlas. I think I heard that they live somewhere in Arizona."

The two of them poured over the map of Arizona and sure enough, there was the Hopi Reservation. They looked closer.

"There it is! Second Mesa! Look, it's a village on the Hopi reservation! Next weekend we're gonna go to Second Mesa!"

Friday came around, the other secretaries at the office were out sick, and Glenda felt she couldn't take the time off to go to Second Mesa. She was crushed. Her husband tried to cheer her up. "I'll tell you what, dear, we'll go for a drive in the foothills. Maybe we can find some Indians for you up there."

They drove to the foothills. Seeing a sign—"Native American Art Gallery"—they stopped and went in to admire the paintings. After a few minutes the attendant walked straight up to Glenda. With no introduction, he said to her, "I've got a great-aunt. She is very old and very wise. Her name is So-and-so. She is a full-blooded Hopi Indian, and she lives in Arizona on the reservation in a little village called Second Mesa. You should go see her." He turned on his heel and walked off.

As far as I know, Glenda still hasn't visited her wise old grandmother. It is worth mentioning, though, that Grandmother Mountain Mahogany is just about the only one of my plant friends who makes her home both in California and in Hopiland.

This story shows how plant medicine connects us to the spirit of place, which is to say, the spirit of nature. The connection with nature is exhilarating and beautiful, but it is not a luxury. Connection with nature is health; health is life. Without it we shrivel and die like the artist with leukemia. With it we prosper. This is so because we are nature; we are made of dirt, rain, sunshine, minerals and gases. How we relate to the landscape within is how we relate to the landscape without. Eating disorders and erosion of the topsoil are part of the same problem. Ecological crisis is a medical syndrome writ large. The plants already know this. They have never forgotten that the fortune of one is the fortune of all, and that is why they are generous and compassionate with humankind.

It is 1988. I have just moved to the Sierra foothills in Northern California, and I am getting to know the plant communities here. I make a dream journey to meet the spirit of the fragrant California Incense Cedar. She is a beautiful brown-skinned woman who lets me know that wherever she grows, the cedar spirit is the mother of every creature who lives in the forest. "The cedars are pleased with you," she says, "and we help you to have success with the other plant spirits. We continue to help you because of your kindness to us long ago."

"My kindness to you?" I say. "When have I ever been kind to you? Aren't we meeting now for the first time?"

"It was my cousin, the Northern White Cedar," she says. "Don't you recall?'

Suddenly I do recall a scene that has been forgotten for eighteen years. It is early spring in Northern Vermont and I am on my way to the cedar bog to cut fence posts....

Spirit

As I write this, my youngest child is two years old. She can barely speak, yet being with her brings me fulfillment beyond what I feel with my articulate friends. There is something special about her. In her presence I am happier, sweeter and wiser. If you have ever loved a child, even for just a moment, you know what I mean.

That special something about my daughter is what I call spirit. Do you remember those moments when you were most in touch with your spirit? It might have happened any time: looking into the eyes of a loved one, watching a beautiful sunset, facing danger, even just washing the dishes. Suddenly, you were filled with peace and energy. Life was full of deep meaning. You were, for a while, fully alive.

Chances are when you were very young, you lived in the fullness of spirit most of the time, just as my daughter does now. If you are an adult, chances are that nowadays these experiences are rare enough to be memorable. What happened to you?

Somehow your heart was broken, or you became insecure, or your self-esteem was shattered, or you were smitten by fear or anger. These terrible events, whatever they were, wounded your spirit.

If you recognize this and admit it to yourself, then you are exceptionally honest. Most of us start lying to ourselves as soon as the spirit starts to suffer. We lie to ourselves about our spiritual wounds because they hurt so much. Physical and mental pain cannot compare to the pain of losing the thing that makes life worth living. This pain is unbearable, so we cover it with anything we can, such as work, food, power, possessions, sex, romance, religion or alcohol. The high from the addiction feeds the lie that we are okay and masks our spiritual pain. We further bolster the lie by lavishing attention on our bodies and minds. Our children have all the luxuries of food, shelter, medical care and recreation, and they receive every conceivable form of education and therapy, but amid this affluence no one confronts the appalling, dangerous poverty of spirit. A leading cause of middle-class teenage death in the United States is suicide.

Cancer, heart disease and drug addiction are minor concerns compared to the problem of spiritual illness. This is all the more true since these symptoms, and most others, are usually disguised forms of spiritual pain. (Adults are not as direct as children—we choose more complicated forms of suicide.)

Technological advances in medicine have not reduced human suffering. On the contrary, wealth and technology have impoverished our spiritual life. We desperately, urgently, need medicine for the spirit, and this kind of medicine does not depend on anything money can buy, as my first encounter with the Huichol people taught me:

I have heard that in Mexico's Western Sierra Madre there lives a great Huichol Indian shaman, one who was taught by a sacred plant to heal the human spirit. His name is Matsuwa, Don José Ríos. It has taken me a year to locate Don José and travel to his home to meet him. Now I am at the end of my journey. As I round a bend in the trail, his hamlet comes into view: children, dogs, pigs and chickens are wandering among a handful of huts made of sticks, with thatch roofs and dirt floors.

I enter the settlement and am led to Don José's hut. Here at last is the great man: a skinny, toothless, unshaven old Indian, dressed in a shabby shirt and ancient, crumbling trousers held up by a piece of twine around the waist. If this person walked by me on the street, I would not even notice him were it not for the fact that his right arm is amputated above the elbow.

Don José welcomes my companions and me. To make us feel at ease, he tells a story: "Last year an American girl came to visit. Her name was Margarita. Ay, that Margarita! She came up to me one day and said, 'Don José, I'm going to give you a massage!' I said, 'Alright.' She said, 'O.K., take your clothes off!' I said, 'NO!' Ay, that Margarita!"

Don José laughs. I wait for the story to continue, but that's it. Evidently this is the funniest thing that has happened all year—the old man can't stop laughing.

During the first hour of my visit, Don José tells the story of Margarita six times, laughing just as hard each time. Obviously I have arrived here too late. The old man is senile.

The next morning begins the ceremony Don José is to lead. I have been told this is a ceremony for the young children. Since they are not yet strong enough to make pilgrimage to the remote mountains, caves and springs where the gods live, the shaman will make a journey in spirit to these places, singing his adventures as he goes. Supposedly his chant will bring the souls of the children along with him so that they may be uplifted by the deities living there.

The old man takes a seat between his two assistants next to an elaborate altar. The children and their parents are sitting on the ground, rattles in hand, waiting for the spiritual voyage to begin. Don José spits out the stub of his cigarette and begins to sing in the Huichol language. The drummer picks up the rhythm, the children join in with their rattles and the assistants chant the refrains.

All day long the children sit under the hot sun, rattling accompaniment to the shaman's song. Just yesterday they appeared to be normal, active, healthy children, and normal children do not sit still unless they are fascinated by something. I have to admit that in the cracks between my boredom and stiffness, I myself have been having colorful visions of various landscapes. I wonder what the children are seeing. Could it be that the ceremony is working, that Don José is taking their spirits to meet the gods?

It is late afternoon now, and the first day of chanting will soon be over. Someone tells me that the shaman is singing about the rain god. I notice a change in the light and I look around. There are enormous black rainclouds over the mountains. A lightning bolt strikes a nearby peak, and thunder rolls. Within moments a rainstorm surrounds us. The village itself remains calm; the sun is still shining here. Don José sings on. After twenty minutes or so, his chant draws to a close. Everyone gets up, stretches, and strolls home. As soon as all are safe in their huts, the storm closes in and drenches the village.

The next day the children once again shake their rattles as the shaman sings from morning until evening under clear skies. Again a rainstorm suddenly appears in the surrounding mountains. As before, the storm closes in on the village only after Don José concludes the ceremony and everyone is safe indoors.

A few days later, I approach Don José and ask him to perform a healing on me.

"What's your problem, sonny?" he asks.

"I've got hay fever."

"What's that?"

"You know...allergies."

"Never heard of them."

"Well, sometimes my eyes get itchy and my nose runs and I sneeze a lot."

"All right, come by my house in the morning."

The next morning I present myself at his hut. He shoos away a couple of hens and welcomes me inside. He produces one of the few items of furniture in the hamlet—a low milking stool—and seats me on it. He stands in front of me, staring silently. At length he pronounces his diagnosis of the cause of my hay fever.

"You've got a girlfriend on the side, huh?"

"No, Don José, I haven't been with any one else since I've been married."

After his performance in the ceremony, I began to think maybe he wasn't senile after all, but now I am sure he has lost it. I have never been unfaithful to my wife.

"Nope, you've got a girlfriend on the side. Sorry, sonny, don't mean to offend you; I'm just telling you what I'm seeing.... Hey, you are a serious case! Your pistol is about to drop off!"

With this he turns around, strides over to the wall, and reaches into a basket. He produces a small wooden wand with feathers tied to it. He approaches me and makes passes around my body with the feathers, accompanied by popping sounds made with his lips. From time to time, he puts one end of the wand on my body and places the other end to his mouth, sucking and slurping loudly. Then he makes a disgusted face and spits onto the floor a glob of what looks like thick brown mucus. He once again remarks on what a difficult case I am. He tosses the wand back into the basket and tells me to return the following day.

I notice no effect whatsoever from his treatment, but the next morning I dutifully return to his home where I am treated to the same routine as the day before. This time he seems satisfied with his work. He draws himself up to his full height and declares, "There! You're clean!" He returns the wand to the basket and then wheels around. "You're going to remember me now, sonny! You're going to remember me for the rest of your life!" He strides out of the hut.

Once again I notice no effect. I am dejected. I have come all this way for nothing. Tomorrow I start my journey back home.

When nighttime comes I can't sleep. I am lying on the ground wide awake, unable to ignore the fleas and cockroaches feasting on my body. Don José's words come to mind: "You have a girlfriend on the side." For the first time I admit to myself that in a hidden corner of my heart I never let go of the lover I had before I met my wife. That lover has been inside me, gnawing like a worm in an apple.

"Your pistol is about to drop off." An overstatement, maybe, but for sure this situation has been robbing some of my sexual energy. Well, okay, a lot of my sexual energy. How did the old guy know this?

"Now you are clean!" That is exactly how I feel! Somehow Don José has sucked all the crap out of me. I feel as clear and energetic as a baby. My heart fills with love for my wife.

Two days later when I reach home, I am still full of love. My wife receives me at the door. She looks into my eyes and knows the ghost is gone. In this moment we wed.

With the power he received dreaming with a plant, this illiterate Indian has healed my spirit and brought me to wholeness. Despite his poverty, he has given me a great treasure.

Years later I found out that it is not necessary to be poor, illiterate, or Indian in order to learn deep healing from a plant—most plants will teach anyone who is interested. If you have the interest, follow up on it and see for yourself.

As a way to begin your apprenticeship with plant spirits, feel free to try the following technique. It may not turn you into as great a healer as Don José—that depends on whether you are as great an apprentice as he was—but my students and I have performed many healings with the power we acquired with the following method:

Put yourself in an open and receptive state. Consider this: the mind is not subtle enough to grasp spirit or make judgments about it. How can we know what is possible? The spirit that moves through a plant might have compassion for you and take a form your mind can understand. Before you go any further, thank the plant spirits in advance for their help and hospitality. Do it aloud. This will help open you, and the spirits will like it.

Keep thankfulness in your heart as you assemble the following materials:

- a drum and someone to beat it for you (If these are not available, then a Walkman-type cassette player with a shamanic drumming tape will work fine.)
- a small amount of loose tobacco or cornmeal
- a reliable, easy-to-use field guide on the flora of your area
- a notebook and pen (Colored pencils or magic markers are also a good idea.)
- anything else that helps you feel empowered

Go for a walk outdoors at a time and place where there are many different kinds of wild plants growing. Wander with no destination in mind. When you come across a stand of plants that are especially attractive to you, approach them. Speaking aloud, introduce yourself by name, and explain that you have come to learn from the spirit of this species. Thank the plant for summoning you and for any help it may be willing to give. Since you are asking for a gift, it is only good manners to offer one in return: sprinkle the plants with a little tobacco or cornmeal.

Now turn to your field guide and identify the plant to which you are speaking. (Identification is usually possible only when the plant is flowering.) Make sure the plant is not poisonous. If you have even a slight doubt about its identity, have it confirmed by a qualified botanist. There are deadly poisonous plants growing in almost every locale.

Study the plant closely. Try to memorize the shapes, colors and geometry. Make a drawing of the plant. Observe what kind of soil it grows in, what kind of light it likes, and how it relates to other plants, insects and animals. Smell the different parts of the plant and then, asking its permission and forgiveness, carefully taste a tiny bit of the flowers, leaves and root, provided they are not poisonous.

Now that you are familiar with the plant, begin to connect with it. Be still. Take your time. Become the plant. Experience the world around you as the plant does. At this point you may be flooded with images, feelings or information. After you return to normal consciousness, jot down your experiences in your notebook.

Return to a quiet and comfortable indoor space. You will need a monotonous steady drumbeat of two to four cycles per second, so prepare your drummer or your tape player. Make yourself as comfortable as possible. (For most people, this means lying on your back with a pillow under your neck and/or your knees.) Close your eyes. Take a few deep breaths, relaxing more deeply with each one. Affirm your intention of meeting and learning from the spirit of the plant you are studying. Start the drumming.

With your eyes still closed, visualize yourself entering a hole in the earth such as a cave, a spring or an animal hole. Once inside the hole, you will find a tunnel leading downwards. Go down the tunnel. Immediately, or after some time, you will see a light at the end of the tunnel: follow it. Move out of the tunnel and into the light. At this point you will have entered a different realm—the dream world of shamanism. (If you don't succeed the first time, be patient. Entering the dream world takes practice.)

You may need to take a few moments to accustom yourself to the dream world. If you feel vague or distracted, remind yourself of your intention and then carry on. People or animals may offer to help you; feel free to accept any offers that feel good to you. Once you feel confident, start looking for the plant you have come here to meet.

When you have located the plant growing in the dream world, look around. You will find a life form associated with the plant. It might be a person, an imaginary figure, an insect, an animal, even a light or a disembodied voice. Whatever it is, this is the form the plant spirit is taking in order to communicate with you. Approach the spirit and introduce yourself. Explain that you have come to learn, and ask if you may learn from this plant or use it in some way. If the reply is positive, then ask the spirit to teach you.

The teachings of plants come in many forms. The spirit may give you a classroom-style lecture. If so, listen intently so as to remember every detail. More often the transmission comes in a non-verbal form. You may find yourself being swept into an exotic adventure. You may simply find that you experience intense emotions. In every case the key is to remain attentive. Once you ask your question, whatever happens is part of the answer.

When you feel your dream is complete, return to the plant spirit and thank it for its help. Ask if there is any way you can repay its kindness, then take your leave. Signal your drummer to give you a more rapid drumbeat. Quickly retrace your route, go up the tunnel, out of the hole, and return to your body. Take a few minutes of silence to mentally review what happened in your dream.

Slowly get up and record in your notebook every detail of your experience. Be complete and precise. No matter how vivid the dream, details will vanish from your memory over time unless they are written down.

Now is the time to start interpreting the dream material. Your dream may be self-explanatory or it may require a lot of thought and contemplation. Some dreams yield their meaning only after they are illuminated by strange coincidences that take place later. This can take months or even years. Be patient.

Some time ago I was teaching a group of people in Central California to dream with the spirits in this manner. We had dreamed to meet our personal guides to non-ordinary reality, and the people in the group were sharing their experiences. One young woman, Paula, said she had met the historical Indian woman, Pocahontas, whom she called "Mother." The dream material seemed satisfying to me, but as she recounted it, Paula's tone of voice sounded disappointed, even sarcastic. I questioned her about it.

"Well," Paula said, "I grew up on a very remote farm in North Dakota. There weren't any real kids around to play with, so I played with imaginary friends. My main companion throughout my childhood was Mother Pocahontas. So, obviously, I'm just making this up, right?"

I thought that Paula's childhood relationship with the spirit of Pocahontas only made the dream more credible. I suggested that she return to Mother in her next dream and ask for some sign that their friendship was real and not just imaginary. She agreed. After the next session, Paula reported that Pocahontas had been waiting for her when she arrived. She had offered Paula a ring as a token of love. The ring would appear in ordinary reality and then Paula would know that Mother really was her teacher. Paula was not to go looking for the ring; it would come to her.

In her dream, Paula had studied the ring closely and now she recounted what the stones were, how they were cut, and all the details of the setting. As Paula had extended her hands to receive the gift, she had noticed that her wedding ring was missing and it was precisely on the ring finger of her left hand that Mother had placed the dream ring. What, she wondered, could be the significance of this? The entire experience was curious to her, and not entirely convincing.

Some time after this class was over, I moved to Northern California. A year went by. I forgot about Paula and Pocahontas. Then one day I got a letter. Paula wanted to let me know about some things that had happened since the class:

> The first thing happened only a couple of months after you were here. I was walking by a jewelry store in San Luis, and I saw a ring that was very similar to the one Mother had given me in my dream. I got real excited and was just about to go in and buy it, but I realized that it wasn't exactly the same. Anyway, she had told me not to go looking for it, that it would come to me, so I passed it by. The next strange thing was only two weeks ago— I lost my wedding ring! I still can't explain how it happened. I never took that ring off, not to do the dishes or shower or anything. I just looked at my hand one day and it wasn't there! I was so upset. Michael and the kids and I scoured the house and the car. I retraced my steps to the Safeway. I even went so far as to rent a metal detector and go over every inch of the yard, but no good— it was gone!
>
> After that, just last week, I got a letter from my old friend Karen in Tucson. I hadn't heard from her in about seven years. Anyway, in the letter Karen said that she still thinks about me a lot. In fact, just a few days before, she was walking past a jewelry store and she saw a ring in the window, and she just knew that it was mine, so she went in and bought it for me. There was this little package in the letter. I opened it up and it was *the ring!* Exactly, down to the tiniest detail! I was amazed! I had

to try it on immediately.... There was only one finger that it fit on: the ring finger on my left hand!

I thought you would enjoy hearing about all this. I guess I've changed my mind about Mother. Thanks a lot for the workshop.

In addition to dreaming and psychotropic substances, there is a third way of learning how to heal the spirit—the way of pilgrimage. Some locations are the home of tutelary spirits, and under the right circumstances a visit to one of these sacred sites can bring about a spiritual transformation. The training of most healers and seers involves at least one such experience: Moses on the mountain, Mohammed in the desert, and Jesus in the River Jordan are illustrious examples. The birth of plant spirit medicine a few days after my first pilgrimage is a much less illustrious example from my own experience.

There are many ways to perform spiritual pilgrimage, but the elements of sacrifice, exertion and fasting are common. The idea is to put yourself in a difficult or dangerous situation with no recourse other than the spiritual power you are courting. Each site has its own etiquette, worked out between the local people and the spirit of the place. These protocols are practical and effective, but not always easy to come by. In some places the native people are not willing to share this information with outsiders, and their reluctance must be respected. In other areas the knowledge of the power places has been lost.

I think it is quite ethical to use the abandoned power places of tribal people. In fact, the spirits of such places are often lonely for human attention, since they achieve their own greatness by conferring greatness upon their devotees. One can use the dreaming method to contact the spirits of these places and ask how they would like to be approached. Often prayer and intuition also work well, as they did for me on a pilgrimage to an abandoned power spot in the Sierra Nevada. The following is an account of the decisions I faced on that journey.

The sweet, benevolent power of this mountain captivated me from the moment I saw it jutting above the trees. I have climbed it in a kind of happy trance. Now I put a tobacco offering in a niche at the foot of a granite outcropping. Suddenly, I am sure I am not the first person to have done so. My trance deepens.

When I return to a normal state, I take in my surroundings more critically. A logging road encircles the base of this peak. Every few minutes a truck clanks by, hauling the carcass of a magnificent old-growth Ponderosa pine. An infernal whooshing sound is coming from the valley on the far side of the mountain. I check it out. The noise comes from a green U. S. Forest Service jet helicopter. It is ferrying logs from a steep clear-cut to a log yard by the side of the road. Watching the government-subsidized rape of the ancient forest, I fall into another trance; this one brings not joy, but nausea.

At last I snap out of it and check the position of the sun. The whole morning has gone by. The mountain is still radiating peace and blessings. The loggers are still at their fiendish work in the valley below. I feel I am being torn apart. One thing seems clear, though. I can't stay in this place. I put on my pack and head down the mountain.

After a few hundred yards, I re-enter the remnants of the forest. I wander into an area where an almost perfect circle of young trees has sprung up around a little meadow. The granite peak is radiant between the pine pillars of this woodhenge. Maybe I should stay here after all.

My mind quickly becomes a morass of indecision: To stay or not to stay? I talk myself into one position, then the other, then the first again. My head is beginning to ache. A sudden clear thought: I don't know what to do, and I'll never be able to figure it out! I turn toward the mountain and get down on my knees. "Do you want me to stay here with you?" I ask. "Help me to know what to do! Please send me a sign!"

Over the ridge of the mountain, a redtail hawk comes soaring in my direction. As he approaches, he suddenly drops altitude; he is soaring just over the treetops now. He glides up to the edge of the clearing, circles around the rim of trees, and soars back in the direction of the peak. I thank the mountain and set up camp.

Two rich days follow. I had planned to stay for three, but suddenly I'm feeling it's time to go. Am I headtripping myself? As soon as the question arises, I'm down on my knees again asking for another sign. Once again a redtail appears, only this time it's a juvenile. He's coming out of the Northeast and flying hard towards my clearing. He comes up to the circle of trees, lights for an instant on a branch over my head, and flies off towards my home. I thank the peak one last time, pack my things, and head for the Jeep.

As I arrive at home; the telephone rings. It is my eight-year-old son calling from the Northeast. It is his birthday today.

Pilgrimage is unreliable. You can do everything right according to the book and nothing may happen. If something does happen, you never know what it might be. We approach the spirits with some request only to find they have something else in mind for us. On the other hand, pilgrimage has this advantage: if you ever receive the grace of a spirit on one of these outings, your life will never be the same again.

For a healer, the purpose of both pilgrimage and dreaming is to acquire medicine for the spirit. Spirit medicine comes from spirit itself; we don't control it or even understand it. Humility is the way.

If spirit ever asks you to do something to help someone, do it. If you do, a miracle will happen. If you don't, you will spend the rest of your life wondering, "Am I making this up?"

Medicine and Dreams

A voice wakes me from a pleasant dream: "Eliot, telephone call for you." I check my watch. It is five A.M. I check my surroundings. I am at a retreat center in southern Washington.

The call is from an acupuncturist friend in London. He is treating Martha, an acquaintance of mine. Martha is in crisis. She has been wild and desperate, holding a butcher knife to her breast for several hours. Now she is in an autistic state and is unable to speak or move. My friend has tried everything he knows and is unable to reach her. He wants to know if there is anything I can do to help.

I assure my friend I will try my best. I return to bed, put on my earphones, and let the sound of the drum move me into a dream of the smiling Huichol Indian and the little deer—the magic of the wind tree. As I arrive at El Picacho, the Indian greets me warmly and asks why I have come. I explain the situation. "Come with me," he says. "I want to show you something."

The wind tree spirits and I find ourselves standing in front of Martha. Behind her stands a masonry wall about five feet high and three feet thick. It runs to the horizon in a straight line. The deer leaps to the top of the wall, the Huichol scrambles up behind him, and I follow. The three of us start walking. As we walk, the man explains, "Someone has the intention to harm Martha. His intention is as strong and direct as this wall. As a matter of fact," he smiles, "this wall is the intention of the malefactor. This person hired someone to hurt the girl by magical means. Although the sorcerer has never met Martha and does not know where she lives, he knows very well how to locate the intention of his client. Therefore, he merely followed the wall in order to locate his victim. But the wall has two ends, not just one, and when we reach the other end, you will discover who is causing this trouble. We will take care of him."

"What about the sorcerer?" I ask. "Don't we need to deal with him, too?"

"The sorcerer is just a professional doing a job," the little man replies. "He has no particular interest in the girl. Now that he has performed his service and collected his fee, he will forget about her."

At length, the wind tree spirits and I arrive at the far end of the wall of intention. There stands Martha's father. I have met this man before in my dreams. He is an ambitious politician in a small Caribbean country. Martha, his illegitimate daughter by a white Irish woman, is an embarrassment to him and a detriment to his career. This is not the first time he has hired a sorcerer to get her out of his way.

The little deer trots over to the father, rears up, and rests his forepaws on the man's shoulders. Delicately, with affection, the animal licks the man's face—his cheeks, his forehead, his closed eyes, his nose, chin and lips. The man's expression softens. A tear trickles down his cheek. He begins to sob softly.

I ask him, "What do you want, my friend? What did you think you could accomplish by eliminating your daughter?"

"All I ever wanted was a little bit of security, of stability, something I could count on in my life," he cries.

I produce a shimmering golden globe, place it in my palm, and hold it out to him. Its effulgence is captivating. I place the globe in his heart. "When you feel in need, look to this sphere in your heart," I tell him. He seems very content with his gift. The masonry wall vanishes. The father thanks me. I thank my friends, the spirits of the wind tree, and return to my bed in Washington. It is eleven minutes past five o'clock.

Later that day I receive a phone call from Martha. She is walking, talking and feeling quite normal. She thanks me profusely for my help. She wants to know what was wrong with her.

"It was your father again." I say. "Have you been in touch with him lately?"

"Yes."

"How long ago?"

"About three weeks ago. I rang to tell him that I was feeling much better and to invite him to my graduation."

"When did you start feeling unwell?"

"A few days after I rang him."

"Listen, Martha, I think your father will be feeling better and won't have to do these things anymore, but let's not tempt fate! Avoid all contact with him. And especially, never let him know that you are doing well. Don't give him any reason to feel threatened by you, okay?"

"Alright."

A man in Washington dreams of a tree in Mexico and a woman in London is healed. What explanation could there be for these bizarre events?

To answer this question we need to look closely at the nature of dreams. Recall one of your most vivid nighttime dreams and remember how real it was. Dreams have all the characteristics of reality: convincing sights, smells, sound, touch; powerful emotional content; even the ability to create effects in the "real" world. It is not uncommon for men to ejaculate while asleep, for example, and people have been known to die of heart attacks during traumatic dreams. There may be different rules in particular dreams, such as being able to fly or perform other unusual feats. Nevertheless, the dream world has a consistent structure, just as the waking world does. The differences between dreams and waking are difficult to pinpoint, yet we generally feel that dream objects are "made up," while in daily life we accept "real" objects made of "solid matter."

There is a story of a wealthy and powerful king in ancient India that illustrates this point. It goes as follows:

> One day the king of the land was reclining on his favorite couch, being fanned by slaves while a handmaiden massaged his feet. He had just eaten a meal of the finest delicacies, and despite the spectacle of the musicians and beautiful dancing girls before him, he became drowsy and fell asleep.
>
> In his slumber the king dreamed he was a miserable beggar wandering along a country road. He had not eaten for several days and when he came across a mango tree laden with ripe fruit, he could not resist the temptation. Just as he was stuffing mangoes into his bag, the farmer appeared with a stick in his hand and gave the beggar a ferocious beating. The sting of the stick on his back made the beggar cry out in pain, and the noise of his own pitiful cries awoke him. Once again he was the great king in his palace being pampered with every luxury.
>
> The king was soon comforted by his attendants and fell asleep once more. Again he assumed the identity of the hungry beggar, again he picked the mangoes, again he knew the farmer's stick, again he cried out in pain and woke himself to his courtly life. This time the king was very upset. It was quite some time before he managed to fall asleep, but when he did, it was only to relive the painful experience for a third time.

When he awoke this time, the king was beyond con-
solation. "Who am I really?" he called out, "A beggar, or
a king? Which of these two worlds is the real one?"

None of the courtiers dared hazard an answer to the
question. In frustration, the king declared that all the
philosophers of his kingdom should appear before him.
Whoever could answer his question would be richly re-
warded, but he who should fail would be cast into prison.

Most of the intelligentsia of that land were soon wasting away in the royal dungeon, but finally a wise one resolved the king's question. He was a young boy who
had been an object of scorn due to his grotesque appearance. His response to the king was that neither the
dream nor the waking experience was real.

Modern science makes the same point in a less poetic way. Research reveals matter to be empty space with a few tiny particles in it.
The particles are energy phenomena. There is no "stuff" in the universe; it is all made out of energy.

As quantum physics explores the nature of energy, some fascinating qualities come to light. For example, in observing a "particle," it is
impossible to determine both its momentum and its location at the
same time because the very act of observing a characteristic causes it to
leap out of the probable state and become actual. All other characteristics are still merely probabilities at that moment. To put this another
way, energy has certain tendencies. The moment we look for one of
those tendencies, it manifests itself, while all other tendencies remain
latent. This is a bit like getting to know a person. If you are provoking
someone's anger, their tendency to express affection cannot be observed at the same time. One might say that energy knows when it is
being watched and it behaves to fulfill our expectations. Energy responds to us. It is conscious.

According to modern physics, although our world appears real
and solid, it is actually an insubstantial realm whose features shift according to the psyche of the person who is observing it. A few para-
graphs ago we described dream worlds the same way. Thus the young
sage's explanation to the monarch: the palace splendors and the farmer's stick were both illusions—made of the same stuff.

The dream of waking life appears to be longer lived, or at least
more repetitive than our nighttime dreams. In actuality, though, all
dreams are timeless. When I was an anthropology student I read the ac-

count of an ethnographer who had spent considerable time among Australian aborigines. He had heard stories of the tracking skills of one particular hunter; the stories were so incredible that he was certain they were fraudulent. When he finally met the tracker, he challenged him to follow the trail of a long trek he had made with another aborigine years before. He was certain this was impossible and that no trail could remain after such a long time. The tracker was happy to take up the challenge, though, and the moment he was shown the starting point, he took off at a trot and ran the whole course of the journey without even pausing to examine the spoor. The anthropologist was humbled and apologetic. He asked the aborigine how he had accomplished this feat. "It was easy," the tracker replied. "I just went back to the time you made the journey and I ran alongside you."

Nighttime dreams from the past also remain available indefinitely. I teach students how to re-enter nighttime dreams, and most people do this easily once they know how.

These anecdotes serve to illustrate that dreams—including the dream of waking life—exist outside the flow of time.

Another interesting characteristic of dreams is that they are permeable and they overlap. One dream interpenetrates another, and a dreamer can move freely among his own dreams and those of others. A woman with three daughters recently told me that she shared a dream with two of her daughters one night. The dream accurately foretold a mysterious life-threatening illness that befell the third daughter in India.

One of the games I like to play with my students goes like this: One member of the class describes a favorite location in the dream world. That student then enters his or her dream, goes to the described location, and prepares some surprises for the others. A few minutes later the others also enter dream reality, find the first student, and discover the surprises waiting for them. Then everyone returns to ordinary reality. The first student writes down on a piece of paper an account of the surprises he or she prepared. The paper is folded and kept from view as each person describes his or her experience. After all the stories have been told, the first student unfolds the paper and reads the initial account. The object of the game is to demonstrate that we can enter someone else's dream. Invariably, some students get all the surprises "right," most get a few of them, and everybody gets at least one.

Most forms of shamanic healing use the timelessness and porousness of dreams to enable the shaman to make his diagnosis. In soul restoration, for example, I teach practitioners to enter the dream of the patient's life and find those past traumatic experiences that caused a part of the soul to dissociate. We then track down the dissociated part and re-integrate it into the life of the soul. (See chapter eleven.) Our patients are astonished to find that we can track long-ago, faraway events in their private lives, but this is easy for us; like the Australian Aborigine, we simply enter the dream of their life and run the course alongside them.

Modern science and ancient wisdom concur, then, in describing our world as a dream—a tissue of appearances made of energy and consciousness.

I am convinced that the universe is a very complicated dream. In order to create it and keep it going, God the Dreamer dreams a multitude of lesser dreamers. Each of these lesser dreamers, or gods, is in charge of dreaming up one part of the world. For example, the stone god has a long dream that brings the stones into being, and when the rain god dreams of showers, the rains fall. Their dreams overlap, and the stones get wet.

Human beings are like gods—we ourselves are dreamers. As time goes on we live more and more within our own dreams and less and less within the dream of nature. This is hard to see. The fish does not see the water and the Los Angeleno does not see the smog. Nevertheless, it is very important that we come to know the difference between the human dream and the dream of nature, or else we will never understand medicine.

One of the fundaments of modern life is the dream of time as a mechanical procession of discreet uniform units. In this dream, seconds click by in single file from an unknowable future through a fleeting present into the jaws of an irretrievable past. Virtually all humankind has agreed on this view, making possible a regimentation of human effort that was unthinkable before hours, minutes and seconds were dreamed up. Clock time makes factories possible.

By contrast, Australian aborigines traditionally live not by clock time, but by what is called the "dreamtime." The dreamtime is a timeless mythic realm in which the Ancestors sing into existence every feature of the natural world. For those who live by the dreamtime, the world is sacred and inviolable. Not a single pebble must be disturbed from its place. The people of the dreamtime will never produce a laptop computer, but they will never produce ecological crisis either.

The Western dream of time is dualistic in that it divides the web of existence into two irreconcilable parts: the present, which is real, and the non-present, which is not real. According to this scheme, the Aboriginal tracker's feat is impossible and absurd since an event cannot occur simultaneously in the past and the present. I give thanks to that

Australian and his anthropologist friend for gently suggesting where the absurdity truly lies.

Dualism is the proto-dream underlying clock time and all our modern dreaming. Dualism might be defined as the illusion that there are two discreet principles in the universe: self and other. Dualism implies isolation, conflict and a continuous struggle of opposing forces. For this reason, actions based on dualisitic vision are simplistic, aggressive and destructive. For example, a farmer dreams that his livestock is part of "self" and predators are "other." Immediately there is conflict, and the conflict suggests a simple, aggressive solution: destroy the predators. This is precisely the solution humanity has adopted over the past few thousand years. Since dualism is blind to complexity, we have failed to notice that in destroying predators we have disrupted the ecosystem in such a way as to impoverish productive lands and turn them into deserts. (For an in-depth look at this process, see Alan Savory's profound and fascinating book, *Holistic Resource Management*, Island Press, 1988.) The dualistic dream engenders an endless procession of conflict, aggression and destruction as each "solution" creates new problems to be attacked. One who lives in the dream of dualism lives in a battlefield, as a walk through any city will attest.

In the Dreamer's dream of nature there is no duality, no separation into self and other, no conflict, aggression or destruction. In the dream of nature, when a predator kills and eats an animal, it is not "us" against "them." In nature all are "us." A slow, sick or injured animal is provided to predators for the benefit of all. The health of the herd is maintained as the predator feeds its family. The dream of nature is a complex web of mutuality in which each part supports the other.

This is the most important difference between the dream of man and the dream of nature: nature dreams of unity and bliss, while man dreams of isolation and violence. Humans need unity and bliss to maintain their health of spirit. The dualistic dream starves the spirit and gives rise to the gamut of illnesses of body and soul. The job of medicine, then, is to nourish the spirit by bringing people into the source of well-being—the dream of nature.

Nature is dreamed by the gods. The gods are dreamed by God. To commune with nature is to commune with the divine, so healing is truly a religious rite with healer as priest. Humankind acknowledges the link between medicine and religion by giving doctors priestly status. This is true even in our society where the reigning deity, Dualistic Technology, is attended by white-robed initiates.

Despite the robes, however, a practitioner who works within the dualistic dream can only accomplish dualistic goals. For example, a person consults a doctor about a respiratory infection. Immediately it is "us"—the physician and the patient—against "them"—the microorganisms in the patient's lungs. As usual, the analysis implies a simplistic and violent solution: kill "them." An antibiotic is prescribed and the microorganisms are destroyed. But each dualistic solution creates imbalance and so provokes new problems. In this case, the antibiotic has disturbed the patient's inner ecology. A superinfection of yeast organisms emerges in her vagina. Fungicide, another dualistic weapon, is applied, creating further destruction and making the patient vulnerable to the return of the lung infection. A stronger antibiotic is prescribed. The warfare rages on.

There is a more helpful way: The same patient consults me with the same complaint. I know there is no "them" to fight against. It's all "us" trying to work through something for the benefit of this woman. What is trying to be worked through here? I speak with the woman and find she has stifled her grief over the death of her sister. What should have been discharged through weeping has lodged in her lungs and made her susceptible to infection. Why has she stifled her grief? She suffers under the illusion that she is weak and worthless. She secretly fears that if she allowed her grief to surface, she would dissolve in the tide of her tears.

Just as the stones are dreamed into existence by the stone god, and the rain by the rain god, so each plant is dreamed into being by the god or spirit of the species. I have entered the dreams of many plants, and now I select one who dreams of inner strength. I ask the spirit of this plant to include my patient in its dreaming. Immediately the woman notices a feeling of peace, accompanied by ineffable sadness. Without knowing why, she bursts into tears.

By the time she reaches home she is weeping uncontrollably. This continues for two days, interrupted only by spasms of coughing which produce thick, old mucus. By the time the weeping stops, her respiratory infection has cleared. More important, she now enters a rich new experience of herself and her life.

Several years ago my left shoulder joint suddenly froze and became painful. There was no apparent cause for this affliction, and each of the healers I consulted failed to affect it. One evening it occurred to me to ask one of my plant spirit allies for help with this condition. The spirit's response was to tell me I had to move out of Santa Barbara. I loved Santa Barbara. I had made my home there for many years and I was not eager to leave. At the very least I wanted an explanation. I argued with the plant to no avail. At length I relented and assured it I would move. Instantly my shoulder got fifty percent better. That gave me the conviction I needed to uproot my family and start a new life in an unfamiliar place.

It took about a year to accomplish the move. Just after we arrived in Northern California, my father came down with a terminal illness. Since I now lived relatively close to him, I was able to attend to him, heal our strained relationship, and be with him at the moment of his death. In addition, after we left Santa Barbara a ferocious fire, whipped by eighty-mile-per-hour winds, swept through the canyon where we had lived, destroying our former home and seven hundred other houses. One person lost her life in that blaze. Her remains were found in the creek bed beside the ruins of our house. When I moved north my shoulder was completely healed, but that was incidental.

Frozen shoulder, lung infection, whatever the complaint is, it's always the same thing: something beneficial trying to happen. In true medicine there is no conflict, no enemy, no disease, only the opportunity to bring someone out of the dream of strife into the dream of wholeness.

There are many medicines to help a person enter the dream of wholeness. Although plants are well suited to the task, it is not necessary to use them. Two things are necessary, however. First, the medicine must be non-dualistic. Second, the medicine must have the power of dreams. A practitioner does not acquire this power by accident. Lofty, well-focused intention is required, and intention must be married to knowledge and skill.

Some systems of medicine, like Flower Essence Therapy devised by Dr. Bach, are strong in their intention to uplift the spirit, but weak in their knowledge of how to do so. By contrast, conventional Western medicine is a Hercules of knowledge and skill, but defaults completely on intention. In fact, technological medicine deliberately sets out to remove intention from the healing encounter. Modern pharmaceuticals are "clinically proven" by the double-blind study, wherein researchers determine whether symptoms are removed when neither the physician nor the patient knows whether a drug or an inert placebo has been administered. I have a nickname for the double-blind study. I call it "the blind studying the blind." Intention provides the vision by which the patient finds his way out of the dream of illness. When intention is removed by the double-blind method, there is no healing left to study—only the empty husk known as "absence of symptoms." Since there is no model of health in Western medicine, the method flounders without a goal to apply itself to.

By now you may have a pretty good idea why a man in Washington dreaming of a tree in Mexico may very well heal a woman in London. The dream world is not limited by time or space, and plants in particular access the source of healing, the divine dream of nature. In order to arrive at this understanding, in this first section of the book we have examined the four components of plant spirit medicine dreams, namely plants, spirit, medicine and dreams. Along the way, we have considered shamanism, pilgrimage, Native American and Native Australian philosophies, and the nature of humans, time and reality. We have seen the goal of this form of healing and have understood there is a method to help reach that goal.

After all this, we can finally answer the question "Am I making this up?" with a resounding "Yes and no." No, I am not making up what the plant spirits give me or what they do for my patients, and yes, I am making up most of the rest of my life.

Part II

My Plant Spirit
Dream

An Ordinary Life

I was born in Chicago and grew up in Winnipeg and San Francisco. My father worked as a manager for various small businesses, and my stepmother was a housewife. My upbringing was conventional in every respect, down to the divorce of my parents when I was eight years old. As a youngster I was sickly and intellectual and had no feeling of kinship with nature. In fact, my allergies to pollen led me to dread plants as the enemy.

While a graduate student in filmmaking during the late 1960s, one day I realized that I knew nothing about the earth I lived on. It suddenly seemed urgent that I find out, so I left the university for a farm in Vermont. On the farm my ignorance led me into one problem after another, but I enjoyed farm life nevertheless. I found a satisfying lesson in each new difficulty. Especially satisfying were my experiences with herbal medicine.

I started practicing herbalism because of a cranky old goat named Eloise. When Eloise got an eye infection one day, I took her to a veterinarian who pronounced there was no cure for her. He assured me she was going to die, but offered a prescription anyway. I thanked him, took the prescription, and left. When I got home I tossed the prescription into the trash and decided that since the vet couldn't help, I might as well try to treat her myself. I looked up her ailment in a book of veterinary herbalism. The recommended herbs were growing on my farm, so I picked them and dosed her according to the instructions. Within a few days she was her normal self again. Her disease had completely disappeared.

After a few more successes, I discovered I had a passion for natural healing and I wanted to make a profession of it. In order to do so I needed a teacher, but I had no idea how to go about finding a teacher, or whether such a person actually existed. One day my neighbors in Vermont told me about their friend Diane, who had contracted a mysterious disease in Asia and traveled extensively trying to find someone who could heal her. Everywhere she went she heard stories of a great acupuncturist named J. R. Worsley. Since none of the practitioners she consulted had been able to help, she went to consult Worsley at his home in England. The Englishman quickly removed Diane's illness and brought her to a wonderful state of health she had never experienced before. Diane was so impressed that she stayed on to study with Professor Worsley.

This story gave me faith that the kind of teacher I needed did exist after all and that I would surely find him. I left the farm to start looking. Three years and many disappointments later, I finally did find my first teacher. He turned out to be none other than J. R. Worsley himself! I first heard Worsley speak at a seminar. He was teaching about the Chinese medical tradition of the Five Elements, and he was simultaneously funny, down-to-earth and profound. His medicine affirmed everything I had learned on the farm and promised to teach everything I wanted to know. I forgot about my local weeds and went to England to learn what I could about acupuncture.

Chinese medicine, as I discovered, attributes healing to the balance of natural energies. In classical times Chinese physicians placed great emphasis on the mind and spirit, and today Dr. Worsley still teaches that these realms are within the province of acupuncture. In keeping with tradition, he holds that the earth and its creatures are made of the same energy that turns the wheel of the seasons. In fact, he says, the seasons mold human nature. Each of the Five Elements corresponds to a season and the energies of these seasons nurture and sustain us in different ways.

Hot summertime energy shows up in the structures that maintain our temperature: sweat glands, heart, circulatory system and the metabolic fire in each cell. Physical survival depends on the right amount of heat, and heat is also essential to our minds. When we "warm up" to others, we know joy. Our spirit thrives on the warmth and joy that give meaning to life.

Indian summer is the fifth or "extra" season. At this time of year, Mother Nature offers a sweet bountiful harvest that provides food for the body, understanding for the mind, and a spirit that responds with sympathy to the needs of others. Nourishment is prepared and delivered by the stomach, spleen/pancreas and breasts.

As the old year wanes in autumn the crisp air announces the beginning of something new. The lungs take in fresh inspiration and guidance while the colon gets rid of feces along with grudges, hurts, sorrows and feelings of unworthiness. Autumn teaches us to value what we have and to grieve for what we have lost.

Winter is a time of inner quiet that puts us at the wellspring of will and ambition. While nature sleeps, the rain and snow fill earth's reservoirs with water, the fluid of life. Our kidneys and bladder control the fluids that keep body, mind and spirit flowing. Winter enables us to know fear and awe.

Spring is a burst into the future, a time for creatures to take birth and grow. This time is not over when our bodies reach full stature. We must keep growing all our lives, or else we become stunted, frustrated and angry. The organizers of our growth are the liver and gall bladder.

The five seasonal energies are the Five Elements, the stuff of which everyone and everything is made. Classical Chinese medicine teaches that the balance of these energies is health, and imbalance is illness. The goal of healing is to restore natural harmony. When this is done, symptoms will disappear automatically since they are only messengers of imbalance.

Chinese medicine notes that the state of a person's elements can be detected by observing the emotions. There are several ways to detect a person's emotions. An animal can tell precisely how a person is feeling by noting their scent, and as a student of acupuncture I learned to recover the use of my nose so that I too could smell people's feelings. Emotions also have color. I learned to perceive the subtle but distinct hue that each emotion lends to the complexion. Emotions make sound. When we are feeling sympathetic, for example, our voices become quite musical, whereas when we are angry, we make harsher sounds. Infants who do not yet understand words are able to interpret the sound of the voice perfectly well, but as an adult I had to re-sensitize myself to this instinct. Emotions throb with the heartbeat. Following classical Chinese medical procedure, I learned to feel the arterial pulse in twelve different locations, and this gave me detailed information about the balance of the elements.

Professor Worsley also educated me in the ways of the spirit. On one occasion, he spent a classroom week talking about the spirit, and on the last day he offered an experience of what he had been talking about. One by one, he invited each student to come to the front of the class and receive acupuncture treatment for the spirit. Before long one man was laughing uncontrollably, while another was slumped in a corner with a dazed look on his face. A young woman was chuckling happily as tears streamed down her face, and another was sobbing and screaming. Dr. Worsley's needles had touched the spirit of each student, and each had been transformed by the experience.

When the Professor needled me, I felt rivulets of sparkling energy flowing through my body. After the feeling wore off, I did not notice any further change. I reflected on the acupuncture points he had used on me and I recalled that those points were useful for mending energies shattered by trauma. This puzzled me, because I was in love and there were no traumas in sight at that time. The next day I flew home, and my loved one greeted me with the news that our affair was over. This caused me great pain, but I was not shattered by the blow since I had already been treated for it.

In England I began to appreciate how nature fulfills human life. I saw that when nature is out of balance, we feel a longing that drives everything about us, including our thoughts, feelings, tastes, cravings, voice, skin color and odor. Most importantly, longing distorts our experience of life. Our symptoms merely dramatize the true disease, the need of our soul.

I returned to the United States in 1976, full of enthusiasm and ready to bring summer sun, harvest sweetness, autumn inspiration, winter peace, and the rebirth of spring into the hearts of my patients through acupuncture, and I have maintained my practice from that time to this.

During the early years I thought a lot about Professor Worsley's teaching on herbalism, which he used to deliver in one sentence: "Anything that can be done with needles can also be done with herbs, but if you use herbs, for God's sake use local ones, because they are not ten times stronger, they are not a hundred times stronger, they are *one thousand times stronger* than plants that grow someplace else." I liked this teaching. I did not know why local plants are stronger, and I had no idea how plants could heal the spirit. Dr. Worsley didn't have a clue either. I believe he was speaking purely from intuition, and my intuition told me he was right.

In July of 1980, after a year teaching at Worsley's College of Traditional Acupuncture in England, I was on an airplane returning to California. Somewhere over Canada's Northwest Territories I made a promise to myself: "I am going to revive the use of local plants to heal the spirit." It was a rash pledge. I had nothing to support it with except youthful idealism, but since I was youthful and idealistic, I took it seriously.

Arriving in Santa Barbara, I began to search for sources of information about medicinal uses of local wild plants. Herbal literature was no help because it was based on European and East Coast American plants. Inquiries with local Native American people were also fruitless since Chumash herbal lore had nearly disappeared as a result of cultural genocide.

With no outside authorities to turn to, I resolved to use my own mind. Chinese Medicine provided me with a set of correspondences which I decided to apply to plants in order to figure out their properties. For example, Indian Summer energy gives rise to the yellow color, the sweet taste, and the stomach's capacity for digestion. The first plant I considered was common fennel, *foeniculum vulgare.* This plant puts out yellow flowers in Indian Summer. Every part of it is intensely sweet and it has a reputation as a tonic to the stomach and digestion. My analytical method was a great success with fennel since this plant was obviously saturated with Indian Summer energy. If this was the first success of my analytical method, though, it was also the last. Every other plant I studied had a mishmash of conflicting correspondences; the color corresponded to one season, the taste to a second, the time of its appearance to a third. It became clear I was not going to get what I wanted this way and I didn't know how to fulfill my pledge. I needed a new approach, and since I had no idea of what that might be, I decided to shelve the whole project.

By this time I had made my first visit to Don José Ríos (Matsuwa), the Huichol Indian shaman in Mexico. The experience, as I recounted in chapter three of this book, made a deep impression on me. I sensed that learning more about shamanism might help me with my work, but I did not know any practical way of getting shamanic training.

Within a few months I was approached by Carolyn Carr, an acquaintance of mine who wanted acupuncture treatment for some health problems. Instead of money, she proposed to pay by teaching me something she thought I would find interesting. I barely knew Carolyn and had no idea what she wanted to teach, but I instinctively accepted her offer. I soon confirmed that my instinct was accurate. As a young girl, Carolyn had discovered she could leave her body and journey beyond limitations of time and space, acquiring knowledge and power as she went. In a word, Carolyn was a shaman (although at the time, neither she nor I knew that label applied to her). In any case, this learning to journey among the dream worlds was the "something" she thought I would find interesting. I worked with her for about a year, deepening my knowledge of acupuncture and exploring other areas of interest to both of us. It never occurred to me to apply this method to learning about plants.

After Carolyn and I parted company, I still had a yen to learn something about "shamanism." I heard that the American anthropologist Michael Harner was teaching basic shamanic technique in a weekend course, so I traveled to New York to study with him. I was delighted to find out that my year with Carolyn had already given me a bit of experience in shamanism. I was also happy with Michael's course. It was clear he had more to teach, so I signed up for further study.

It was Michael who suggested a technique for contacting plant spirits that was precisely the new approach I needed to fulfill my pledge. English plantain, the first plant I contacted, assured me the plant spirits would be happy to teach me and had, in fact, been waiting for almost two hundred years in the hope someone would ask for their help in healing the human spirit.

After that first contact, I took advantage of every spare hour to learn from the plants of my region. I had already learned their language—the language of the five seasons. The plant spirits gave me knowledge I could immediately put into practice and put it into practice I did, gingerly at first, but with more confidence as I saw evidence that it worked. Within a few months, I had amassed a body of plant lore that would have taken generations to acquire any other way.

While I have been blessed with exceptional teachers, my story is unexceptional in every other way. I have no unusual talents, no mystical powers. I had a middle-class childhood with the usual amount of suffering and insecurities. I was trained by my parents only in the rational materialism of the day, and I was not initiated into any Native American tradition. Over the years I have come to honor my ordinariness and to consider it a testament to what can be accomplished by a person with no resources other than a sincere interest in healing.

Fire

The sun, thin and weak with age, has finished its short journey across the sky. Underfoot, ice crystals grow amid blackened stems. The few remaining birds have tucked their heads under their wings...there is nothing to sing about. Among all the creatures, only the People are happy and talkative. The icy blackness does not penetrate the circle of their campfire where they sit sharing the adventures of the day. They rejoice in good fortune and laugh off the bad, for they have the pleasure of shared warmth.

Young mothers are tucking in their babies. The bigger children sit at Storyteller's knees, eagerly awaiting one of his tales.

Storyteller looks at the expectant little faces. He chuckles. He places two logs on the fire. "Thank you, older brothers," he says.

One of the children raises her voice. "Storyteller, why do you always talk to the firewood and call it 'older brother'?"

The adults laugh. They know this question is sure to be answered with the story of "Why the Sun Has To Rest at Night." This is a complicated tale involving some of Storyteller's best characters: Bear, Trout and Blackberry Bush.

The story begins and continues into the night, punctuated by giggles and guffaws. One by one the children drop off to sleep, and when the telling is over, Storyteller allows himself a few last chuckles as he banks the fire. His wife approaches, wiping tears of laughter from her cheeks. She smiles an invitation to him. In her eyes, he sees the glowing red coals.

In this scenario the campfire gathered the people, warmed them, and brought out their mirth. The campfire came from the sun. It was stored in the flesh of plants.

We receive our energy by eating the sunlight in plants and animals. Every heartbeat and every step you took today was fueled by the sun. Each of your cells is like a tribe gathered around its metabolic campfire. The fire keeps people from dying of cold and also brings the gifts of laughter and conviviality.

Outside, leaves orient themselves to the sun. Inside, cells orient themselves to the heart, the internal sun radiating through the bloodstream. What is a warm-hearted person? A cold-hearted person? These are more than figures of speech. It is the sun shining on our soul that makes us feel pleasure, joy and compassion.

Recently I was consulted by a fifty-year-old man whose heart had been out in the cold for so many years he could no longer find the enthusiasm to do anything. He just collected unemployment and puttered around the house amid a clutter of unfinished projects. I gave this man a plant spirit to warm him and give him the heart to take the helm of his life once more. His face flushed pink. The next day he phoned to say he was burning up and he hadn't stopped crying since the night before. Was there anything I could do to turn down the heat? I assured him both the heat and the sadness would soon pass and he would feel much better afterwards.

He phoned again the following day with new enthusiasm in his voice. He had some things to talk to me about and invited me to meet for dinner. His chat over dinner was full of purpose and vigor. The day before he had taken the steps to close a major business deal that had been blocked for months. He had also phoned the nearby university with instructions on how to bring to fruition one of his inventions that had been languishing in the laboratory for years. The invention, significantly, consisted of an instrument and surgical technique to clear out blockages in the arteries of the heart.

The heart and the sun were worshipped in old religions. According to modern science, the sun is radioactive gas and the heart is a muscle. We have abandoned ancient wisdom in favor of scientific superstition, and heart attacks, nearly unheard of only one hundred years ago, have become one of the greatest causes of death in our society.

Actually, many heart attacks are caused not by the heart itself but by a failure of the "heart protector." Ancient Chinese physicians likened the heart to an enlightened Emperor, the embodiment of love on earth. The Emperor controls all the activities of the empire of body-mind-spirit but is not up to the shocks, insults and intrigues of rough-and-tumble life on the streets. Thus, the Emperor has a special minister called the Heart Protector. The heart protector keeps us from "taking things to heart." When this minister is strong, we laugh things off and keep our joy intact. When the heart protector is weakened, we suffer excruciating vulnerability, mistrust and bitterness.

The heart protector function does not correspond to an organ. You can not point it out in a cadaver. For this reason, conventional medical doctors are unlikely to take it seriously. Nevertheless, it is as real as the nose on your face. Maybe it's more real, since you can't go to a plastic surgeon and get a heart protector job!

Ralfee Finn, now a practitioner of plant spirit medicine, had a particularly vivid experience of what can happen when the heart protector gets the warmth it needs after years of deprivation:

> I was skeptical before I started treatment. I had no idea what to expect, but when I received the first tincture I instantly dropped into a deep state of consciousness, and I saw a spirit in front of me. I knew it was a plant spirit.[1] At the second tincture, I heard Chopin playing. It was as if he were present in the room, as if I were inside the piano. It was so beautiful! When you gave me the third drop, an angel appeared to me. I felt great. I felt a lot of energy move up into my chest. That night I had important dreams.
>
> I felt elated for about fourteen hours and then the work of cleaning things out started. On a physical level, I had to poop constantly for days. That was okay, but the emotional work was pretty devastating. I started to go through my characteristic hurt behavior. You asked me to demonstrate something in front of class, and I couldn't do it. I was overwhelmed by old feelings: not being good enough, being betrayed, being ostracized from the group, not being part of the group, retreating inside to some place where I "knew better, anyway." This exacerbated not belonging. Since it's "better" not to belong, let's stay not belonging. Even though I was experiencing this, I was also watching it. I knew I had felt like this all my life. I was getting to my deepest symptoms of "aloneness" and sorrow.
>
> I went through hell for twelve hours. I had all of the worst memories from my life: the alienation and betrayal in the music business, the hurt I went through when I left my spiritual community and seventy-five of my

---

1. Note: Several months later, I introduced Ralfee and her class to a plant known as "bleeding heart." We made a dream journey to meet the spirit of the plant. Afterwards, Ralfee told me I must have given her bleeding heart in her first treatment, since the spirit she met was clearly the same one that came to her at that time. I consulted my treatment notes. She was right. —E. C.

closest friends never even called to find out why I wasn't there any more. As a child I went through that all the time. I was never able to belong. There were times that night when I even felt like killing myself. It's strange to say this, but I feel I was able to move through this quickly because the treatment was sustaining me somehow.

The next day in class we made a dream journey to Fire. When I got to the heart protector I saw a huge open wound just ripped apart.[2]

I began to piece together that this wound was a spiritual wound: not belonging, not feeling that I could trust. It had been repeated over and over in my life. My cynicism, my criticalness—I could see that these were my defenses, my protection from the pain of not belonging.

On the third day I had the courage to state to the class what I was feeling. This was a big leap of trust. It enabled me to belong. I wouldn't have been able to do that before.

Since then I've noticed dramatic differences. I'm able to go into new situations. When we got back from the plant spirit medicine class I went to the first meeting of a dance class I had signed up for. When I arrived, there were about a hundred people there. I panicked. "This is too many people! Let's get out of here!" But I was able to stay, participate, and even enjoy the class. I know that for some people this would be insignificant, but for me it was a really big deal to feel protected enough to participate like that.

I've been to L. A. and New York; I just feel totally at ease wherever I go. With each treatment I feel a vital essence is being restored to me. Each time it strengthens a little more. It's a little easier to trust. Also, I've become sexually interested again for the first time in years—a big difference! Here's another thing: I never have to wear blush anymore. Everyone thinks my skin looks radiant. No one in New York can believe that I'm not wearing makeup. I'm glowing from the inside out.

---

2. This corresponds with my assessment of Ralfee's condition at the time.—E. C.

I'm much less self-conscious about my body. Years of therapy about body image have not been as fruitful as a few plant spirit medicine treatments. It's not so much that my body is changing, although I have lost weight. It's more that I have a buoyancy, a resilience inside, so that life doesn't feel despairing. I know that I'll never have to go through that despair again. Now I have more vitality and more ability to do what I want to do.

It's not as if you get treated by a plant spirit and immediately you drop thirty pounds, although I suppose that could happen. It's as if the care and nurturing that you're looking for in whatever your drug is—whether it's food or shopping or alcohol—you're getting that from the inside now.

At the time of the summer solstice, the sun's longest journey across the sky, there is a huge festival in Santa Barbara, California. At noon a parade starts down the main street which is lined by everyone in town who isn't in the parade itself. The parade is dedicated to the sun, to summer, and most of all to fun. The goal of each float is to make people happy. Outlandish costumes, grotesque monsters, ten-foot-tall clowns, samba dancers on stilts, jugglers on roller skates, block-long serpents, pantomime artists and jazzy bands heighten the festivity. When the parade is over, the participants and spectators walk to a nearby park where they spend the rest of the day feasting and dancing.

Santa Barbara's Solstice Festival is entirely non-commercial. No one gets paid for the huge tasks of organizing and preparing for the event. Why is this so unusual? The answer has to do with fire, sex and spirit.

"Come on, baby, light my fire." It doesn't take much subtlety to get the connection between fire and sex; fire is what gives us pleasure. Let's have a quick look at how we are doing with respect to sexual warmth. On the physical level, we are plagued with problems. Impotence, frigidity and premature ejaculation cause marital strains. Among the unmarried, teen and preteen pregnancy and sexually transmitted diseases are huge problems. If we are enjoying sexual pleasure at all, it seems it is only with the wrong people at the wrong times. On the mental level men, women and children are teased without mercy. Sex sells alcohol, cigarettes, coffee, milk, automobile tires, electronic equipment, vinyl siding and more.

We are looking for the hot stuff because our spirits are cold. Did our parents and teachers make it their job to warm our spirits? Most likely, the people who did are the ones who now stand out in our memories. We have only one institution that even recognizes the human spirit and that is the church, but our churches are dour and solemn. Where are our temples of divine laughter?

What brings warmth and pleasure to our spirit? No amount of sleeping around can do it. Romance doesn't do it either. Bombing Baghdad didn't help. The only thing that can warm us is love. We live in a cold-hearted society. We are spiritually frigid and so we have an infantile craving for pleasure. This craving is whipped to a frenzy by purveyors of merchandise of every kind. For this reason, Santa Barbara's Solstice Festival is unusual. If we had a healthier relationship to the sun, every town in the nation might have innocent non-commercial celebrations.

Observing the action of the sun on growing plants, the ancient Chinese maintained that fire has the power to bring things to maturity. A mature human being is one whose spirit has been warmed by the fire of love.

People from mature societies like the Hopi have some penetrating observations about our own culture. Fred Coyote tells the story of an anthropologist who came to a Hopi elder to record some of his people's songs. The old man took him out on the edge of the mesa and he sang a song. The "anthro" was recording and making notes and he said, "What is that song about?"

The old man said, "Well, that's about when the kachinas came down into the mountains and then the thunderheads built up around the San Francisco peaks and then we sing and those clouds come out across the desert and it rains on the gardens and we have food for our children."

And the old man sang him another song. And the "anthro" said, "What was that song about?"

The old man answered, "That song was about when my wife goes down to the sacred spring to get water to prepare food for us and to prepare the medicines because without that sacred spring we wouldn't live very long."

And so it went all afternoon. Every time the old man would sing a song, the "anthro" would say, "What's that about?" And the old man would explain it. It's about something or other—a river, rain, water.

Eventually this anthropologist was getting a little short-tempered. He said, "Is water all you people sing about down here?"

And the old man said, "Yes." He explained, "For thousands of years in this country we've learned to live here. Because our need for this water is so great to our families and to our people, to our nations, most of our songs are about our greatest need. I listen to a lot of American music. Seems like most American music is about love." He asked, "Is that why? Is that because you don't have very much?"[3]

Adelle was an attractive professional woman of middle years who came to me for plant spirit medicine. She smiled easily and laughed a lot and was successful, well-liked and happily married. Her laughter had a slight edge, but she was so vivacious no one would have guessed she complained of fatigue.

Adelle's voice, emotions, odor and complexion told me what she herself was not yet ready to confide—her fire was burning low. Looking at her face, I noticed a subtle ashen color—a lack of normal healthy ruddiness. (A healthy red color has nothing to do with exposure to the sun. It comes from the flush of joy and pleasure within.) I discreetly sniffed the odor of her body, which smelled scorched—like burnt toast. Laughter predominated in the sound of her voice even as she spoke of unhappy things. She presented herself as a joyful person, but the joy was forced. I inferred that in the past she had been treated with coldness and indifference and had felt unloved and heartbroken. She had been working so hard at appearing cheerful that she had tired herself out.

I invoked the spirit of foothill penstemon for Adelle. Foothill penstemon has a beautiful fuchsia-and-blue flower that makes anyone happier just to look at. The spirit of this plant brings joy but is not a narcotic. It makes you work to clear out heartache. After receiving the penstemon spirit, Adelle closed her eyes and volunteered that she felt a pleasant sensation that appeared "blue and fuschia" in color. I checked her pulses. The response was very good, so I ended the treatment and asked her to return in a week.

After leaving my office nothing unusual happened to Adelle until the next day. Around noon she came down with a fever and flu-like symptoms and went home to bed. She was lying with her eyes closed when she began to relive a long-forgotten scene from many years before. As a teenage girl, she is lying in bed. Her body is covered with painful welts, and she has cramping in her abdomen such as she has never felt before. Suddenly her mother strides into the room, looks at her, and says, "You feel bad because you are about to become a woman, and that's what being a woman is—pain and suffering!" Without another word her mother wheels around and strides out of the room.

---

3. Printed courtesy of The Sun Valley Center for the Arts and Humanities, *I Will Die An Indian*, Institute of the American West, formerly a division of the Sun Valley Center, Sun Valley, Idaho 1980.

Adelle the teenager, and now Adelle the woman, cry brokenheartedly. How could her mother be so cold and indifferent?

Just as the sorrow was beginning to subside, Adelle found herself reliving another moment of heartbreak: the death of her father. This trauma was followed by another and another. In all, Adelle spent three hours in bed weeping. Afterwards she felt shaken, but well enough to get up. The flu symptoms were gone.

In the days that followed she felt extraordinarily well. Colors appeared vivid and intense. Food tasted like ambrosia. Music moved her to tears. Sex was ecstatic. Her relationship with her husband reached new heights. Her complaints about fatigue were completely forgotten; the sun was now shining in her heart.

QUESTIONS: FIRE AND YOU

By answering these questions you can savor your relationship to fire. Relax for a moment by a flame—a candle or sunlight would be fine. Enjoy the blaze, thank it for its presence, and invite it to shed light on the friendship you share. Consider these questions one by one, and address the answers to the fire itself. Feel free to laugh or cry. Say what is in your heart. Contradict yourself if you like. Honest answers are right answers.

1. When was the last time you had a really good laugh?
2. How do you feel in hot weather? Cold weather?
3. Do you go "hot and cold" about people? About things?
4. How do you feel about hot food? Hot music?
5. Do you wear red clothes? Would you buy a red car? Live in a red house?
6. How do you feel about summer?
7. What or who do you feel passionate about?
8. What do you do for fun?
9. When have you felt heartbroken?
10. When have you felt disheartened?
11. When have you felt out of control?
12. When have you tried to control others?
13. Does your work bring you joy?
14. Does your family life bring you joy?
15. When have you felt vulnerable and unprotected?
16. How do you feel at parties?
17. Have you heard any good jokes lately?

18. How is your sex life?
19. What do you do wholeheartedly? Halfheartedly?
20. Do you enjoy being with people?
21. How important is friendship to you?
22. Do you perspire? Easily? With difficulty?
23. Do you have any circulatory problems?
24. How do you feel about being in the sun? Sunny weather? Cloudy weather?
25. When have you dreamed of fire or explosions?
26. Do you like burnt or bitter things like coffee or burnt toast?
27. What do you feel bitter about?
28. Do you feel loved by your partner? Family? Friends? Associates?
29. When have you felt that you would never love again?
30. When have you felt your heart overflowing with love?

After writing down or thinking about your answers, what questions created the most feeling response in you? What questions were difficult or easy to answer? Can you see where your fire, your passion for life, is strong or where it may be weak? Address the flame or sun once again and ask it for understanding to perceive where the passion, the fire of your life, is almost gone, dying away, or where it's at the edge of wanting to blaze forth. Ask the fire inside of you how and where you can burn more intensely and joyfully. Finally, sit quietly and allow yourself to feel both the joy and the heartache about what you see in your fire. These feelings will bring you closer to body heat, mind spark and heart passion: your fire.

Earth

Before I was born, my beautiful dark-brown Mother longed for me. She wanted to feel me suckling at her breast. She waited a long time for my arrival—many centuries, perhaps—until at last she could wait no longer. She removed two lumps of flesh from her own body and modeled them into a young woman and a young man. She made these young people beautiful in each other's eyes, and they joined together to bring forth a child, which was me. At last I had arrived! How happy my beautiful dark-brown Mother was! How contented!

Now that I had arrived, though, there was work to be done, for I was hungry and started crying for something to eat. My Mother caused the hairs of her beautiful dark-brown body to grow green and tall and to bear fruits and seeds. She made these foods beautiful and gave me eyes to feast on their beauty. She made them fragrant and gave me a nose to appreciate their perfume. She made them tasty and gave me a tongue to taste their exquisite flavors. She made them nutritious and gave me a stomach to digest their juices and turn my Mother's flesh into my own.

My beautiful dark-brown Mother knows that if I were to stray from her, I would soon become weak and emaciated. For this reason she keeps me with her, always pressing her body against the soles of my feet. I feel her underneath me, and I know who I am and where I stand.

Since we are together constantly, I am learning from her example. She understands me, and this shows me how to understand others. She feeds me, so I am learning to feel secure and open-handed. She has never abandoned me, so I have learned loyalty. She has never forgotten me, so I have learned how to remember. Perhaps memory is the greatest gift she has given me because it is the only one I can give her in return.

This is your story, too. You and I have the same beautiful dark-brown Mother. Let us give the best thanks a grateful child can offer: "Beautiful dark-brown Mother, we remember You with love."

I am here thanks to many meals eaten by many people. The same could be said of my home, my family, this book and the computer I am writing it on. People and their accomplishments are made of food, and food is born of the soil. Earth is our Mother.

How well do we remember our Mother? Can we recall her 10,000 years of labor to create each inch of soil? Agricultural experts talk of "acceptable rates of erosion," while Midwestern dirt drifts down the Mississippi. Have we forgotten who feeds us? Once we are all finally taken off her breast, who will bring us our food? Where will we get it?

A mother's breasts freely give nourishment, security, identity and fulfillment. Our society hates mother's breasts and does everything it can to keep children away from them, for we have come to believe that nourishment, security, identity and fulfillment should be purchased. Women are no longer solely devoted to motherhood; they are members of the work force, earning money to try to buy the things for their children that only their breasts can really provide.

In many less industrialized societies, mothers know that children need to nurse and to continue nursing, often for two, three or even four years. In such cultures, breasts are openly displayed without shame or provocation. Many of us, on the other hand, have never had our need for the breast fulfilled and so it persists as an obsession in adult life. Our dissatisfaction and rage at not having enough of Mother distorts our fascination. We reject the real, serviceable, sagging maternal breast. It is the idealized virgin breast we crave. Thus such modern inventions as the brassiere, the silicone implant and breast cancer. Thus also the rejection of feminine values such as cooperation, nurturing, intuition and sympathy. Thus the substitution of idealized sterile foods for real ones. And thus, finally, the rape of Mother in all her forms, including soil, forests, wildlife, water, air and the bodies of women.

From our first day to our last we conduct an intimate relationship with Mother Earth through our mouths. As an organ of eating, our mouth is an extension of our stomach, and so our stomach keeps us connected to Earth. Most people nowadays are aware that what goes into the stomach can either support health or tear it down. Are we also aware that the mind has a stomach that must be properly fed? How nutritious was your mental diet today? A well-filled stomach brings contentment, and a contented person is not envious, greedy or competitive. A contented person does not feel superior or inferior and has no need to measure up to others. Contentment brings gratitude and the ability to sympathize. Did your mental diet bring you contentment today? Did you feed yourself on understanding and brotherhood or stress and violence?

These days everyone has a certain amount of stress and violence in their diet, but as long as we don't overindulge, a healthy stomach can churn it, mix it, and rot it down into digestible form. In the same way, the stomach gives us our ability turn an idea or experience over in our mind. In the West, we call this "rumination." In China, they say the stomach gives people the ability to ponder. If the stomach is weak, however, even bland food can be indigestible. Similarly, innocuous experiences are churned over and over in a vain effort to break them down and assimilate them; this is worry and, eventually, obsession.

The pondering, potentially obsessive faculty of the stomach is beautifully expressed in Rodin's famous statue, "The Thinker." It is no coincidence that Rodin was a Frenchman, for the French are known to be stomach-oriented. Witness their obsession with food, particularly food that has been worried over and rotted down, such as ripe cheeses, aged wines and elaborate sauces. The French are constantly chewing something over, and if there is no food at hand an idea will do just fine.

Whether in France or elsewhere, middle-class life offers many opportunities to feed the body and the mind. Physical food is never farther away than the corner convenience store, and with mass media we don't even have to leave our own homes to find food for the mind. But where do we go to find nourishment for our spirit? Are there convenience stores, or any stores at all, that provide food of this kind? The spirit has a stomach that needs to be fed regularly and well. A hungry spirit feels deprived and insecure. It may make an elaborate show of giving to others, but really there is nothing to give. A starving spirit eventually gives up the struggle and resigns itself to slow, wasting death.

Once an old man came to me for help. Since he could not walk he had to be carried into my office. This was not difficult to do, for he weighed no more than sixty-five pounds in his soaking wet diaper. He was placed on my couch. I took his cool hand and welcomed him, but he did not respond to my greeting and instead lay there staring at the wall. The nauseating sweet odor of his body and the dirty yellow color of his complexion made an interview unnecessary, though. Clearly his Earth was impoverished.

I looked at this man sympathetically and asked him only one question: "Do you have an appetite?"

"No," he replied.

I brought him a plant spirit to strengthen the spirit of his stomach. Immediately he turned, looked me in the eye and said, "I could go for some good barbecue right now!"

After a little more chitchat he was ready to leave. Although he moved very slowly and needed two people to help him, he insisted on walking. For the next hour, as I was treating other members of his family, I heard him in the waiting room, complaining loudly: "I'm starving! Let's get out of this place and go get us some barbecue!" At last his family took him to a nearby restaurant where he ate a hearty portion.

Mothers need to be strong. As anyone who has tried it knows, mothering involves a lot of hard work. Within the body the work of mothering is done by the spleen and pancreas, which transport nourishment from the stomach to the cells. It is as if they ran a shipping firm with thousands of yellow trucks delivering glucose to every part of the country. The spleen/pancreas function is dynamic and muscular and enables us to be dynamic and muscular as well. It is another of Mother Earth's gifts and another aspect of her genius; to every creature with a mouth she gives muscles to get food.

This function of bringing the sugar to the cells or bringing the sweetness to life is a deceptively simple one. If modern life more often tastes bitter and metallic, it is because our spleen/pancreas is too ill to do its job. Symptoms of this illness are everywhere; the most obvious one is our addiction to sugar. It is worth noting that table sugar is a machine-made product. Industrial technology makes sugar refining possible and it also creates the need for this addictive substance, since industrialized society produces people who do not know the sweetness of being supported by the earth. Such people are so deprived of sweetness that they will buy it regardless of the cost to their own health. In the world today, the universal artifact of our culture, more widely available than penicillin, gasoline, polyester or rock and roll, is Coca-Cola.

Another symptom of our spleen/pancreas imbalance is our transportation network gone berserk. As we have seen, the function of a healthy transportation system is simply to deliver the goods and services necessary for the support of the people. In our society, however, transportation has become an end in itself. It has long since ceased to be our servant and has instead become our master, exacting heavy tribute through car payments, insurance, parking, garage construction, repair bills, gasoline prices, taxes to support road construction and maintenance, subsidies to transportation industries, and standing armies and military interventions designed to protect access to petroleum. If this weren't enough, our cancerous transportation system has made our air unfit to breathe and our water unfit to drink. It has given us a country where people suffer from ulcers, hypertension, and all manner of other diseases related to the stress of getting to work and back; a country where the hiss and stench of the automobile penetrates every forest and meadow; a country where we don't know how to live without cars and trucks. This is so incredible that it needs to be repeated: *we no longer know how to live without cars and trucks!*

In most temples of transportation—auto parts houses, repair shops, show rooms, truck stops, dispatch offices, warehouses, truck bodies—one finds a little shrine in which is displayed the image of a mythological sacred object. The object it represents was lost long ago, and this primordial loss caused many people to dash madly about trying to find it. This dash was the birth of the modern transportation industry. No one has yet recovered this sacred object, but each man who takes up the search secretly believes he will be the chosen one. The sacred object, of course, is the female breast.

Carolina is a woman who helps my wife with the cooking and cleaning during the week. On weekends her pleasure is to walk to her plot of land in the hills outside of town and tend her corn. In late summer last year the Earth brought forth a bumper crop. Carolina saved her money and bought a small mare to pack in the harvest. The mare doesn't need costly gasoline or repairs. Its wastes enrich rather than pollute the environment. It will eventually pay for itself with its offspring. And there is no need to put pictures of tits on it since it came equipped with real ones of its own.

The Lakota shaman, Wallace Black Elk, was once asked by a sincere young man what we could do to heal the Earth. He replied this way: "We don't have to heal the Earth; she can heal herself. All we have to do is stop making her sick." To this simple truth I would add that the Earth can heal us, too. Despite the neglect and the devastation we have heaped upon her, despite our illness and our ignorance, our Mother still loves her children. She has not turned her back on us yet; her breasts are still full of the milk of sympathy and understanding.

Robert, a physician in his mid-fifties, discovered a way to help his patients heal the pain of their minds and spirits as well as their physical complaints, and he initiated a program in one of the major hospitals in his area. His success aroused the envy and suspicion of his colleagues who did not understand his work. Robert was subjected to humiliation by the hospital bureaucracy and was eventually fired. Around the same time, his wife divorced him and kicked him out of his home. Within a few months, he contracted a serious illness. His doctors diagnosed hepatitis and a large tumor, presumed malignant, in the neck of his pancreas. As a doctor, Robert knew such a cancer is untreatable and fatal, and in a whirlpool of fear and worry, he began to put his affairs in order. His scant strength was fading quickly, as he was unable to eat. Since he could not get up, he called me to his bedside.

Robert told me his story with such desperate attention to detail it took him an hour and a half to recount it. He longed for me to understand, to know, and to fully sympathize with how he was feeling. His longing touched me and showed me his need for his Mother. I summoned Her in the form of a plant spirit and then got up to go. To my surprise, he leapt to his feet and followed me out the door of his bedroom. He proceeded directly to the kitchen, opened the refrigerator, and stood there grazing hungrily as I left the apartment. When I saw him again two weeks later, he was active and confident. Far from being bedridden, he was about to leave for Germany to visit a spiritual teacher who bills herself as an incarnation of the Divine Mother.

QUESTIONS: EARTH AND YOU

By answering these questions you can taste your relationship to Earth. When you are really hungry, take your favorite food to a pleasant place in nature. Give thanks and eat your food slowly. Note how it feels in your mouth and stomach. Pay attention also to how your surroundings make you feel. Consider these questions; chew them, digest them, and answer them from your gut.

1. How do you feel about your mother?
2. How do you feel about your home?
3. What makes you feel secure? Insecure?
4. Do you feel that people understand you?
5. Are you able to nurture others?
6. How do you take care of yourself?
7. Do you care for others at your own expense?
8. How much do you worry?
9. Do you feel you are too fat? Too thin?
10. Do you overeat or eat when you are not hungry? If so, why?
11. Do you eat foods that really satisfy you?
12. Do you enjoy eating?
13. If you are a woman, how do you feel about your breasts? If you are a man, how do you feel about women's breasts?
14. Were you breast-fed? For how long? How do you feel when you watch someone else being breast-fed?

15. Do you enjoy sweets?
16. How is your digestion?
17. What makes you nauseous? What makes you vomit?
18. How do you feel about walking barefooted? Putting your hands in dirt?
19. Would you like to be alone in the wilderness?
20. How do you feel about caring for young children?
21. Would you paint your kitchen yellow? Your living room? Your car?
22. How do you feel in Indian Summer (Harvest Time)?
23. When have you felt that the rug was pulled out from under you?
24. What makes you feel grounded? Ungrounded?
25. What obsessions do you have?
26. How is your memory?
27. Do you have a shoulder to cry on? A sympathetic ear to listen to your problems?
28. How do you know who you are?
29. Do you know where your next meal is coming from?
30. What did you feel grateful for today?

The earth represents the physical, emotional and spiritual nourishment and support that we each need. As you consider your answers, how does the physical world and other people (including yourself) give you basic support? As you have written out or thought about these questions, what were the issues in which your insecurities clustered? What are the things that give you the greatest stability? Go outside and sit on the ground and ask the earth to give you the support and nourishment you need in your life today. Tell this great Nurturer and Stabilizer what you need and then receive it by feeling your body relax and your heart and mind grow calm. Both your security and insecurity bring you close to the one who feeds your flesh, your mind and your soul: Mother Earth.

Metal

The old shaman, Don Guadalupe González Ríos, lead us on a spiritual pilgrimage to the holy land where his gods dwell. We fasted in preparation and went to a sacred spring where the old man anointed us with holy water. After that, he guided us into the wilderness where we confessed our sins, telling Grandfather Fire the name of every sexual partner we ever had. Only then were we pure enough to receive the blessings we sought.

After we entered the hallowed valley, Don Guadalupe built an altar under the open sky. On a whoosh of Eagle's wing, he passed each of us as much of his spiritual power as we had the strength to withstand. He lit and blessed a fire and brought us around it. Then he sat and watched over us as his secret essence did its work. Some of us threw ourselves onto the earth and wept, others trembled with fear or laughed or danced or sang or sat quietly in wonder.

Many hours passed. Night fell. The moon rose and was sung to by the coyotes. We were still in a circle around the fire under the starlit sky. Sensing we were now settled enough to receive his words, the old shaman spoke:

"You have traveled a long way, made a lot of sacrifice to come here, to receive something. I have put my secret into you so you won't say, 'I went to see the great shaman so-and-so and he didn't give me anything.' No, I'm not like some who deny what they know because they don't want to share it. I am going to die some day. What is the use of having learned something if I can't pass it on? I would like everyone to be able to know what I know!

"I want you people to understand that everything I have, I owe to my father. When I was very little, maybe three or four years old, my father carried me on his back up the holy mountain where the wind tree lives. When we got to the summit, he lit candles and left offerings for me. He stayed up all night praying for me. I didn't know what was going on; I just fell asleep. Years later when he asked me if I remembered those journeys, I told him I didn't. He said, 'Of course not! You were asleep most of the time!'

"When I got a little older my father called me to his side and said, 'Listen, my son. I am just a poor Indian. When I die you will not inherit cattle, you will not inherit a house or money. But you will inherit a path of healing and knowledge, a way through life that will sustain you.' I told my father that it was good, that I accepted his gift. 'I am going to give you my heart,' he said. 'You will inherit my heart.' And he put his secret into me.

"From the time I was twelve years old, I didn't bother my father any more; on my own I started making pilgrimages to the mountain. I went every year for six years, and then I maintained my vows for another six. Then I came for six years to this place where we are now sitting, and I maintained my vows for six years after that. By the time I was four or five years into my apprenticeship, I saw that what my father had said was coming to pass. The deer would come and offer themselves to me. And all those who came to be touched by my hand were healed and made well. It was just as he had said it would be.

"At one point I wandered off the path my father had given me. I began looking for a different life. But it went badly for me, and I returned.

"Six years to the mountain, plus another six is twelve. Six years to the desert, plus another six is twelve again, or twenty-four years in all. Then I repeated the whole thing. Forty-eight years and more I have been walking this path of knowledge and healing, and it supports me to this day.

"There have been times when I doubted that my father was even my father. But I know he was my father: he planted the seed of wisdom in me. I owe everything to him. I thank God for my father!

"That is all I want to say to you. Now you know a little bit about the traditions of my people. You speak to me now. Tell me about your traditions."

"Don Guadalupe," I said, "My people have lost our traditions."

"How can this be?" he asked. "The spiritual tradition is fundamental. It is the first thing a person should have."

"With no one to guide us," I replied, "we cannot find the way. That is why we have come from so far to be here with you. None of us had a father like yours to teach us."

"No! Really?" asked the old man.

Betty turned to me, tears glistening in her eyes, and said, "Tell Don Lupe this: Yesterday you told me to confess my 'sins' to Grandfather Fire. I want you to know that the first name on my list was that of my father."

The shaman was stunned by this message. "With his own daughter? Like an animal? How can this be?"

"This is what my people have come to," I told him.

The father is the one who shows us the way through the world; through him, we come to know what is of value in life. His hand on our shoulder gives us the feeling of dignity and self-worth. He is the first and greatest authority. Because he respects us, we respect ourselves; because we respect ourselves, we respect others. Father's role is to recognize our essence, to encourage and instruct us so that it may come forth and bless our life with its unique quality.

Did your father do all that? If so, you are extremely fortunate: your life is rich and your connection to spirit is strong. For you, every mundane experience is important and charged with significance.

Or was your father more like Betty's? He may not have violated your body, but perhaps he violated your soul with neglect. If so, you have suffered great loss and your soul knows depths of grief.

Many of us go around dazed by unspent grief, looking for something to fill the hollow place in our chest. We seek the presence of the Father, our Father who art in heaven. He is the source of spiritual wealth, and if we can't find Him we start looking for substitutes. Often we feel that material wealth will take His place. I need not document how corrosive to the soul this substitution can be. The Huichol Indian Don Guadalupe was as shocked at the poverty of our people as we were at the poverty of his.

Some of us who lack our Father try to compensate by accumulating a wealth of information, facts or learning. Don Guadalupe, who is illiterate, has no book learning to enrich him. He heals people and gives them strength by sharing his spiritual wealth. He does not share it through lecture, since spirit cannot be captured in words. He calls his treasure his "secret." His sharing is a direct act of generosity from one soul to another.

Don Guadalupe used to show a lot of interest in the healing practices of medical doctors. One time, after a particularly profound session of instruction, he expressed satisfaction at my progress. Then he surprised me by asking if I thought a Huichol person would be capable of becoming a medical doctor.

"Of course," I replied. Trying to convey that western medicine requires only a strong intellect, I said, "All that is needed to become a medical doctor is the ability to read very well." Since reading is a mystery to this man, my answer was not at all illuminating. I tried again. "That is to say, Don Guadalupe, that in our medicine there is no secret."

"Ah!" he said. That was the last time I heard him express interest in the subject.

Another way to look for the Father is by accumulating supposed spiritual wealth. Here we find the desperate spiritual seekers who measure their worth by their importance in the sect of their choice, be it religion, therapy, art, science, politics, or even a corporation, police force, or the military. But the collectors of spiritual accolades, like the collectors of knowledge and the collectors of material wealth, don't realize that the Father is not limited to a particular temple. There is nothing special that needs to be accomplished in order to come into His presence. All you have to do is breathe. The Heavenly Father pervades the air around us and enters us through our lungs with every breath.

The essence of the Father is subtle, yet the ancient Chinese referred to it as metal, the densest of the elements. Perhaps this is because metal is the most refined and valuable essence of the earth. In any case, people from many cultures have long accepted metals such as gold and silver as tokens of value. At some point in our history we began to mistake the tokens for the real thing. The result has been centuries of slaughter and exploitation. The lust for a shiny yellow metal drove European people to come to America, massacre its peoples, and destroy the natural environment. This was accomplished thanks to knowledge of steel and with the blessings of a religion that worships God the Father. Lust for gold, allegiance to steel, violence to the spirit, and the cult of a ruthless god: these are the founding values of our nations.

Authority and power are at the core of the masculine principle in men and women alike, yet most of us do not know the difference between authority and suppression, between power and abuse. When was the last time you saw a judge, police officer, professor or your own boss weep while on duty? When did we have a national day of mourning for the people we killed in Iraq, in Vietnam, in Hiroshima or anyplace else? Only recently did the men's movement discover that grief is the key to manhood. This came as a big surprise to many, because grief takes the cutting edge off strength and tempers it with kindness. But when we have been softened and made kind, we are more authentic, more powerful and ultimately, more authoritative.

Grief gets our values straight. It teaches respect. If grief has been deeply felt, a person who has just lost a loved one is clear about what is important and clear about how precious human life is. Our main problem with grief is that we don't really feel it. We think we have to be "strong."

This conventional masculine strength is not really strength at all, but rather a pathological refusal to let go. Before the essence of the Father can inspire us through our lungs, we must be clean, pure and empty inside. This cleanliness is maintained by the colon, which removes filth and brings sparkle, righteousness and receptivity to the body, mind and spirit. There is an old Zen story that could be used to illustrate how the colon and lungs work together. This is my version of that story:

> There once lived a prosperous merchant and his
> younger brother. The merchant had a successful busi-

ness, a large family and a reputation for righteousness. The brother, on the other hand, was a bachelor and a drifter who had never pursued any occupation for long. The merchant was astonished when his brother appeared one day and announced he had married and that his wife was with child. He wanted employment, he said, in order to support his new family, and he begged the older man to give him even the humblest position in his firm.

The merchant was impressed by his sincerity and eagerness, and gladly gave him a job. He was at a loss to account for the sudden transformation in his brother, however, so he questioned him about it.

"Dear brother," the younger man replied, "all my life I have been driven by a desire to know the highest, the most sublime. Agriculture seemed trivial to me, and I was oppressed by the very thought of entering one of the trades or professions. I drifted about, looking for something of value, but my search was in vain, and life seemed pointless and depressing. At length I heard of an elderly man known as Grandfather. He was said to be a man of great wisdom, perhaps even a divine sage. In desperation I decided to go to him to ask for initiation into his cult."

"Yes, I have heard of this man," said the merchant. "Did you visit him? How did he receive you?"

"Indeed I did visit him," said the younger man. "He was practicing the movements of Tai Chi when I arrived. He was as energetic as a man of middle years, despite his great age. After finishing his exercise, he greeted me with kindness and asked me the purpose of my visit.

"'After years of wandering and searching, I have found nothing of value,' I told him. 'Emptiness and sorrow are my lot. I have been told that you possess a great treasure of wisdom, and indeed the sparkle of your eyes and the serenity of your face testify that you have attained something that eludes me still. I have come to request that you teach me.'

"The old man told me, 'It is good that you have come, but I am looking for a disciple who knows how to be receptive. The master, you see, is active, and pours his wisdom into the disciple. It is rather like pouring a cup of tea. Truly your cup is empty and in need of filling. Unfortunately,' he said with a chuckle, 'you have not learned to hold your cup still. If I tried to teach you, my tea would end up being spilled on the table.'

"The interview seemed to have concluded, so I thanked him and took my leave. The old man's words were not lost on me. It was quite true! My quest had led me from one door to the next. I had never stayed with anything very long. No wonder I had been restless and unfulfilled! I decided to change my ways. I married and I intend to stay here in this town, with your help, dear brother."

As years passed, the younger brother worked hard and became a partner in the firm. He seemed to grow ever more ingenious and productive as he prospered. He became a prominent civic leader and one of the most respected figures in his community.

Meanwhile, the other brother was not faring so well. His business still flourished, it is true, but he begrudged his younger brother his high status. Gradually the older man began to doubt himself. He became listless, and his health deteriorated. It happened that he heard of the elderly sage again, and now he resolved to visit him and ask for help. The master had refused to pour his blessings into his brother's teacup because he had been a weak and irresolute young man, but the older brother reasoned that he would be a worthy recipient of the choicest blessings because he had been strong and hardworking all his life. Therefore, he thought, by approaching Grandfather he could find relief from suffering and show up his younger brother all in one stroke.

He journeyed to the abode of the sage and was greeted there with warmth. The master said he had heard of the merchant's reputation and considered himself honored to entertain him. When the merchant explained that he had come to receive teachings, the master seemed very pleased indeed. The sage invited the merchant into his quarters and asked him to share a cup of tea.

"Aha!" thought the merchant. "The symbolic pouring of tea! Just as I thought! I indeed am a worthy disciple! Truly I know how to be receptive, for now the teacher is going to pour his inspiration into me."

The two were seated and the tea set was brought. The host graciously lifted the teapot and began to pour into the cup of his guest, who looked on with a smile of self-congratulations. That smile faded into a look of consternation and then horror as the sage continued to pour. The tea reached the brim of the cup and began spilling onto the table. The host continued smiling and pouring. The puddle of tea on the tabletop widened. When the tea began to run onto the old man's clothing, it became clear that this so-called sage was an impostor, a soft-headed old lout who could not even pour a cup of tea, let alone confer blessings on others. The merchant could contain himself no longer. "Stop, you fool, stop!" he shouted. "Can't you see that my cup is full?"

"Ah," said the sage. "Your cup is so full.... 'I am a great man. I am so clever. I am more worthy than my brother....' How can I pour anything into your cup? It is too full. Your brother's cup was empty when he came to me, and he received total enlightenment three years ago. *Empty your cup.*"

These words dazed and confounded the merchant. All thoughts and opinions were erased, and he became empty. In that state, he was truly a worthy disciple. What more can be said of the wordless moment when a man receives the spirit?

The merchant stayed on and studied under the sage for nine years. At the end of that time he, too, attained enlightenment.

Pauline was a well-educated housewife and entrepreneur of forty years of age. Like most of those who come for help, she started out by telling me her physical problems: "I used to do massage, but my hands started hurting terribly. I went to the doctor, who said I had tendonitis. I stopped doing massage, but I got worse anyway. My hands got weak, no strength in them at all, and the pain was intense. My back started hurting too. A second doctor diagnosed carpal tunnel syndrome, and a third said I had two twisted cervical vertebrae. I took anti-inflammatories and also some natural therapies. I can do whatever I need to do now, but there is still a lot of tension, and it's a real effort to stand up straight.

"I'm having massages done myself now, and for three days after each one I get fever, chills and fatigue. Then I also get headaches, and infections that go into my lungs. I keep having the taste of tobacco in my mouth, even though I quit smoking two years ago. And I still have a cough like the one I had when I had bronchitis years back. Also, my trunk aches, as well as my left wrist and my left knee. If that weren't enough, my bowels are terrible too. I only go once a week."

I drew Pauline out about how she felt in herself: "Sometimes my spirits really aren't that great. I got married a few months ago, and my husband aggravates me. He contradicts me all the time. What a drag! I get kind of depressed. In fact, for the past week I have had zero energy, zero 'oomph.' I'm just exhausted from constantly trying to get going...all the therapies, the massage.... I just feel like giving up. It gets so bad that sometimes I don't want to go on living."

Responding to my question about her childhood, she said, "When I was little I was the apple of my father's eye, but when I was four there was a total break with him, a total rupture. From that time on, the only time he said anything to me was to give me a bawling out for something or other. From thirteen on, I became very rebellious. I know now that I was trying to get some attention from him.

"What happened to cause the rupture with my father? I don't know for sure. I went for hypnosis to try and find out. A memory started coming back...it was vague, but I think there might have been something sexual with him. As soon as this started to come up, these incredible sobs started coming out of me. I cried and cried. Then I blocked the whole thing out, and that is all I know about it."

With Pauline, the white color of her complexion, the weeping tone of her voice, the slightly rotten odor of her body, and the predominant emotion of grief let me know that her suffering was caused by a severed connection with the Heavenly Father. With that understanding, her whole story made sense: The rupture with her physical father plunged the young Pauline into grief that stayed with her, unplumbed, for decades. When she came close to recalling the event as an adult under hypnosis, she wept uncontrollably but did not have the emotional strength to confront it directly. At puberty she started acting out her lack of Father by rebelling against all forms of authority, that is to say, all forms of fathering. Meanwhile the lack of inspiration from the Heavens was slowly making her weaker, resulting in chronic lung problems, chronic colon problems, chronic pain and exhaustion. Only at the age of forty did she come out of her rebellion enough to marry, and the man she chose was hypercritical, just as her father had been. This was the crisis for Pauline. Her pain now went so deep that she no longer wanted to live. At this moment, she was ready to find help.

Help came in the form of a plant spirit that led her back to her Heavenly Father. A week after her first treatment, Pauline's words were: "I feel better. I feel strong, and I have hope." With that hope and that strength Pauline started on the road back to life.

QUESTIONS: METAL AND YOU

By answering these questions you can honor your relationship to Metal. Wake up early in the morning, move your bowels, and go to the summit of a hill or mountain. Breathe deeply. Bow, kneel, or perform a solemn ceremony as a gesture of respect to the experiences of your own life. Take up these questions. Consider each answer to be a gem of priceless wisdom.

1. How do you feel about your father?
2. How do you feel in Autumn?
3. When was the last time you wept?
4. When have you lost someone who was precious to you?
5. When have you lost valuable objects?
6. What golden opportunities have you lost?
7. What do you regret?
8. How are your bowels?
9. What grudges have you held?
10. How important is fresh, clean air to you?
11. Do you feel rich or poor? Why?
12. You have a chance to make a lot of money doing a job you don't believe in. Do you take it? Why?
13. What traditions do you observe? What traditions do you avoid observing? Why?
14. How do you feel around policemen? Bosses? Other authority figures?
15. Does your family respect you? Do your working companions respect you? Do you respect them?
16. What do you do to gain respect?
17. Do others admire you? How do you feel when they tell you they do?
18. Who do you admire? Why?
19. How do you feel at funerals?
20. How do you feel when you make a mistake?
21. When was the last time you admitted making a

mistake?
22. Do you like pungent, spicy foods?
23. Are you an authority on something? Do you enjoy
being an authority?
24. What do you collect?
25. How do you feel wearing white clothes?
26. What are you a purist about?
27. What are your strengths? Your weaknesses?
28. How much metal do you wear?
29. How do you feel around strong men? Weak men?
30. What is your religion or spiritual path?
31. What is the most precious thing in your life?

The energy of Father in all forms of life can wound us, challenge us or anger us. What leads us, sharpens our lives, brings authority and guidance, or gives us riches are mixed together to give us the gains and losses of our life. What in these questions depresses and saddens you? Where in you are the hidden "metallic," steel-like strengths that you need to grow and expand? Go outdoors and breathe deeply. Breath is the source of power that connects us to the Father. Ask this metallic, heavenly power to strengthen and firm your life, to heal loss, welcome opportunity and gain new capability to act and live in the world. Sit now in the center of these feelings and insights and be respectful to the one who breathes life into your body, mind and spirit: your Heavenly Father.

Water

On the summit of a mountain in central Mexico stands a small pyramid known as El Tepozteco. When I first visited it, this monument captured my imagination. What was it used for, I wondered; what gods were worshipped here? I asked friends about it, but they were almost as ignorant as I was. I was told only that the structure was dedicated to two deities: Quetzalcoatl and Tlaloc. These names meant nothing to me, so I decided to find out about the pyramid for myself. I climbed the mountain, scaled the walls, and laid down on the ceremonial platform with some apprehension. Was this where priests with obsidian knives cut the still-beating hearts out of their human victims? Or was it the Incas in Peru who did that? I couldn't recall for sure, so I closed my eyes and hoped for the best.

A jaguar appears. He circles quickly around the pyramid, his tail held straight up. Suddenly he wheels and faces me. "So," he says, "you want to meet Tlaloc, eh?"

"Well, yes, I suppose I would like to meet him," I reply. "How do I do that?"

"I'll take you. Get on my back."

I mount the jaguar. He leaps into the air and bounds upwards. We reach the sky and tear through it as if it were a paper screen. We find ourselves in another, more colorful world under a different sky. The cat continues upward. He tears through this new sky and we enter a third world. He keeps running, tearing through sky after sky.

In the thirteenth world the jaguar comes to a halt and tells me to dismount. As I do so, I look over the edge of the small plain where I find myself. Below me I see the worlds I have just passed through, neatly stacked like the steps of a pyramid.

Turning around, I see a young man with long blonde hair, blue eyes and a halo. His palms are facing forward, and from the center of each palm spurts a stream of water. These streams flow down through the worlds below, eventually forming the waters of our earth, where fish swim and plants flourish.

The young man speaks. "Hello! I'm Tlaloc!"

"You are Tlaloc?"

"Yes."

"Then how come you have blonde hair and blue eyes?"

"You see me as a gringo because you are a gringo. The people who built this pyramid saw me differently. I look different to different folks, but everyone knows me. I am the Rain God."

"It is a privilege to meet you. Please tell me something about yourself."

"You are a student and doctor of the elements," says Tlaloc. "Tell me what you know about rain, about water."

"Have you got a minute?" I ask.

"Sure," replies the deity, taking a seat and lighting a cigarette.

"Okay, here goes—water is sacred and mysterious, the origin of life. I've often wondered why life chose to take birth in the sea. I think the answer is in how responsive water is. The first thing about living creatures is that they move and are still by turns, and water is the element that supports movement and stillness alike. There are so many movements: our joints move in water, our food is digested in water, our sperm swims in water, our brains think in water. The surging of water causes the movements of our souls: the willpower, the ambition. And there is stillness, too. When the water in us comes to rest, we know peace and plunge beneath the surface of appearances. There are eternal moments between breaths, between thoughts."

Suddenly I feel timid giving a lecture to a god. "How am I doing?" I ask.

"Fine!" says Tlaloc, "Keep going."

"Well, the only other thing I want to mention is death. Every living thing seeks life and fears death, so water is both the source of life and the source of fear, as well as courage and awe, which are sublime forms of fear."

"That was very good!" Tlaloc says. "You should be telling people these things! People need to know the things you just said, and more. There is more to say."

"Like what?" I ask.

"Look at the way people squander water. Look how they pollute it. They don't realize they are utterly dependent on rainfall, that water is the very blood in their veins. For most people, water is just a commodity to be bought and sold; something that comes out of a faucet. To them, rain is a nuisance that makes driving inconvenient. They treat me as if I had no feelings. Naturally, I treat them the same way. Diseases, phobias, exhaustion, floods, droughts— what do they expect?"

"And you want me to tell people about this?"

"Yes, tell them. They need to know."

"They won't believe me! I'm not even sure I believe me! Am I actually having this conversation, or am I making it up?"

"You will see," says Tlaloc. "After a while, you will get a sign, a coincidence. This will convince you I am for real. Meanwhile, it has been very nice meeting with you. You may go now."

I thank Tlaloc and ask the jaguar to return me to my world.

Several months later, I visited my sister in California. On her bookshelf a certain volume caught my eye: *Mesoamerican Mythology.* I took the book down and opened it at random. There was a photograph of an Aztec bas-relief. At the top of the carving stood a young man with his hands at his sides, palms facing forward. A stream of water spurted from each palm and flowed into the world below, where fish swam and plants flourished on river banks. The caption read: "Tlaloc, Aztec Rain God." Here was the coincidence I had been promised!

I considered the words of the deity: "They treat me as if I had no feelings." It was true. My patients were polluting their inner waters with all manner of toxic substances. They were using stimulants, they were overworking, depleting their reservoirs of ambition and will, and then they were coming to me with the resultant symptoms: depression, ___ anxiety, fatigue, phobias, arthritis. On a larger scale, we were treating the waters of the earth the same way—polluting them with pesticides, herbicides, heavy metals, nuclear wastes and God knows what else. In my own town, every year local officials were pumping more water out of the ground than rainfall could replenish.

It wasn't always this way for humankind. There was a time—a long, long time—when we knew we are related to Water.

When my sister-in-law went to visit the Tarahumara Indians in Mexico, they were having a serious drought. Their crops, and therefore their lives, were in danger, so the community got together under the guidance of the shamans. They sang and danced to the Rain God all night. At sunrise a thunderstorm drenched the happy dancers.

We can scarcely imagine the communion those Indians must have enjoyed. We may not even believe such a thing is possible, so alienated have we become. Yet this kind of interaction with Water used to be the norm for all humanity. This was how we survived until just yesterday.

It is still possible today. After I met Tlaloc, I made a dream journey to ask for help for the drought we were having. He gave me a ceremony for bringing rain. It required certain props, including a picture of Tlaloc drawn by me and candles made of chocolate. I drew an awkward little cartoon and set about making the candles. The first one turned out well enough to keep a small flame going. After lighting it I absent-mindedly set it down in front of the cartoon. Within fourteen hours an unpredicted storm rolled in and blessed the town with rain. That storm was followed by several others.

There was no need to call on Tlaloc again until the following year, which was also dry. I performed the full ceremony for the first time on February 3, 1987, in Santa Barbara, California. It was a hot day with clear skies. No rain had fallen and none was forecast, but when I awoke the following morning there were tiny craters in the dust. A few raindrops had fallen during the night. The following days were sunny and dry, though, and it seemed to me the ceremony had failed.

I visited the Rain God again on February 8. "What went wrong with the ceremony?" I asked.

"Nothing. I thought it was charming," he replied. "I sent you a sprinkle to let you know you did a good job."

"Is there something more I can do so we can get enough rain this year?"

Tlaloc frowned. "If people get enough rain every year, they take it for granted. They don't learn anything that way."

"But you don't want nature to suffer, do you?" I asked.

"The plants and animals will survive a year of drought and fire. You should be talking to people and telling them what you know rather than wasting your time here with me."

"I don't know if I can do that," I said. "I don't have the confidence. If I don't get another good synchronicity, I'm going to doubt this whole thing again. You've got to send me some serious rain."

"Can you give me another candle?" asked Tlaloc.

"Sure."

"Okay then, you've got a deal."

I lit a chocolate candle and sat down to compose an article about the Rain God. If he was for real it would rain, and I would have to tell people what I knew. If it didn't rain I wouldn't bother to finish the composition.

I started to write at three in the afternoon. A wind came up and clouds thickened. At five thirty it rained for a few seconds. After midnight it started to come down hard and steady. I finished my article and promised Tlaloc I would begin teaching.

A few years later I was living in the Sierra Foothills of Northern California. The country was in the second year of disastrous drought. The previous year I had read a newspaper article about a group of Iowa farmers who pooled their money and hired a Lakota shaman and his troupe of rain-dancers from the Rosebud Reservation in South Dakota. The Indians arrived and performed their ceremony. It rained three days later, as promised. If this could happen in Iowa, it could happen any-where. Farmers everywhere are practical people. Now was the time to demonstrate a practical alternative to treating water as if it had no feel-ings. I would offer rainmaking services to ranchers and farmers. If I was successful, they would pay a fee and agree to make certain changes that would put them on better terms with water. If I was not successful, there would be no charge or obligation.

I presented my scheme to the Rain God. I told him I didn't have the credentials of a Native American medicine man. Before anyone would take me seriously, I needed to produce some undeniable results. I asked him to send enough rain to keep the grass green in my yard throughout the summer—a miracle in that part of the country. He agreed to help but set two conditions. First, I had to understand that this project was only for helping people find a better way to live. It was not to be my personal ego trip. Second, I had to declare my intention in public before we started; if I wasn't willing to risk ridicule, I might as well forget the whole thing. I agreed to his conditions. I took out ads in the local news-papers announcing my project and started performing his ceremony regularly.

It continued to rain through the spring and into the summer. By mid-July the grass was still green under the oaks in my back yard. Meanwhile, crops and livestock were perishing of thirst in the Mid- and Southwest. I felt the time had come to reach out. I renewed contact with Alan Savory of the Center for Holistic Resource Management in Albu-querque. Alan teaches brilliant, unorthodox agricultural management methods. Since his clients are among the world's most open-minded farmers, I asked Alan to present my offer to them.

Alan explained that the major obstacle he faces in his work is pub-lic acceptance. If he went around talking about rainmaking, folks would think for sure he was crazy, so he had to decline to present my offer. Two weeks later, though, he thought better of it. He was giving a seminar in the hardest-hit part of Texas. The ranchers were telling tales of cracked earth, dying cattle and bankruptcy. "Here," he thought to himself, "is a group that has nothing to lose and everything to gain." He presented my offer. Not a single person responded or even acknowl-edged that the offer had been made. They all went on talking as if noth-ing had happened.

The Tlaloc project was to be for the benefit of others, but nobody was ready to benefit from it, so I stopped performing the ceremony. It stopped raining. The grass in my yard turned brown. I was not able to help anyone else, but at least I convinced myself that there is a Rain God who treats us the way we treat him.

We have to meet every moment with the right juices. Danger needs adrenaline, food needs digestive fluid, sex calls for other fluids. Everything juicy is "water" and is pooled by the bladder spirit. Even our energy flows as a fluid and pools there. When the pool is full, we flow with the changes like water does. If the pool runs dry, there is fear, paralysis—no flow.

The kidney spirit harbors deeper mysteries of water. Consider winter, the season of water. A seed sleeps, gestating under the snow in the dark stillness of the earth-womb. Deep within itself it finds the primeval chaos giving birth to the galaxies. It has arrived at the life spring. Drinking here, the seed imbibes the will to live. Its waters have been charged with a force that brings life out of death and being out of nothingness. It will carry this force into the world and it will pass a drop of it through its sexual fluids into its own seeds.

This force, which is harbored by the kidney, cannot be adequately described; we can only point to some of its effects. The Chinese sages said the kidney is the origin and basis of the life force. A Middle-Eastern sage said: "Unless you are born of water and the spirit, you can not enter the Kingdom of God."

Obviously plants do not have kidneys and bladders, but they store fluids and harbor the mysterious life spring just as we do. What is more, they will bring peace to our waters if we ask them to.

Roberta, a woman in her mid-thirties, is an example of someone who benefited from plant spirits' power with water. As I listened to Roberta's complaints during her first visit, I heard the groaning sound of her voice, saw the blue color of her complexion, smelled the putrid aroma of a stagnant pond, sensed the fear that had paralyzed her, and noticed the theme of water imbalance repeat itself in her life story:

> I used to sleep fourteen hours a night, but I can't sleep at all now unless I get a massage. I feel very bad, defeated; I can't go on. There is a hole in my stomach. I have no inner peace, just constant anxiety.
>
> When I was a girl, I was in bed for three years with nephritis, a kidney disease. By the time I was twelve, I was living in a total fantasy world. I would lie in my sickbed and masturbate hour after hour. It wasn't so much for the pleasure of it; I was just trying to escape from anxiety. But anyway, my sexuality got out of control. I've had about eight abortions, I guess. I've lost count. But I feel very guilty about that and afraid of the consequences.

I've always been one to drift with the tides. My boy-friend of the moment always directed things. After I broke up with somebody in Spain I was so depressed I couldn't get out of bed. This healer finally got me up and I went to work. I made tons and tons of money but I pissed it all away. Like I say, I just drift with the tides.

My mother was very possessive, very critical. She was perfect and always pointed out my imperfections. My father just died three months ago and that's when I really lost it. He was almost God to me. A brilliant paint-er, poet, philosopher. On the other hand, he scared the pee out of me too. He was very violent; he used to beat me with his belt. I've lived my whole life in terror of him. And come to think of it, I've been prone to trem-bling ever since I was a little girl.

Now I feel as if I had run out of water. Everything is dry. It's as if my life were a landscape of salt.

I called on a plant spirit to bring the waters of life back to Roberta. At her second visit, she said she was feeling well in the daytime and wanting to be active again. At night she was sleeping more, but was bothered by nightmares of fish. By her third visit she had entered a kind of wintertime hibernation. She was spending her days dreaming and musing in her darkened bedroom. Roberta's fourth visit was to have been yesterday, but I am happy to say she didn't show up. She was out looking for a job.

QUESTIONS: WATER AND YOU
These questions can help you feel the currents of water in your life. Watch the movement of a river and imagine it flowing through your mind. Allow the answers to the questions to flow downstream with no hesitation.

1. How do you feel by the sea? By lakes? Rivers? Swamps?
2. How do you feel in Winter?
3. Are you afraid of the dark?
4. Are you afraid of death?
5. What is your greatest fear?
6. Do you enjoy scary movies?
7. Do you seek danger?
8. How much salt do you want? How much salt do you eat?

9. Do you enjoy drinking water?
10. Are you a good swimmer?
11. What are your ambitions?
12. How do you feel when you have to do something you have never done before?
13. When has fear kept you from doing something you wanted to do?
14. When have you overcome your fears?
15. How do you feel in blue clothes? In a blue room?
16. When have you lost control of your bladder?
17. What or who inspires awe in you?
18. What makes you anxious?
19. What phobias have you had?
20. Do you fear God?
21. When have you felt nervous?
22. When have you felt excited?
23. Do you enjoy roller-coasters and other carnival rides?
24. What motivates you to get out of bed?
25. Do you meditate?
26. When have you trembled?
27. How do you feel in rainy weather?
28. Where does your tap water come from?
29. Where does your sewer water go?
30. How much water did you use today?
31. When have you experienced peace?

As you consider the variety of responses to the questions, think about how wide and deep your emotional responses to life are and how constricted and narrow they are. Where do you feel most frightened? Close your eyes and feel yourself sink into the great river, the great energy flow of life. Ask this lifespring to take you into the depths of life's experience. After you've bathed in this source of your existence, reflect on its gift of quenching your deepest longing, and give thanks that Water will take you to it.

Wood

Some say Dreamer's first dream was the elements. Out of His imagination sprang fire, earth, metal and water, all surging in chaotic flux.
After He finished His creation, Dreamer contemplated it and was
pleased...for a while. Eventually, He got bored with the flux. Although it is
pretty intriguing compared to sheer nothingness, flux hasn't got much of a
plot. In fact, with no here or there, no before or after, no you or me, one could
say that flux has no plot at all. So it was that Dreamer began to long for some
good stories to wile away the eons. This is remarkable considering stories
hadn't been invented yet, and there was no one to tell them or act them out, but
then Dreamer is a remarkable Person.

One of Dreamer's many remarkable qualities is inventiveness, and He invented a way to generate a neverending supply of really terrific tales: He
dreamed a tree growing right at the center of his centerless universe.

Maybe you are thinking that a tree isn't much as a source of epic dramas,
but things were different back then at the beginning, and so the entertainment
industry really does owe it all to a vegetable. Here is how it happened: Once
the tree was growing, it needed room to grow. Zap! Suddenly space existed
where only chaos reigned before. And if this weren't enough, the tree needed
its limbs to grow up and its roots to grow down. Zap again! Suddenly there
was direction in the universe. Now that there was a way to get organized, the
tree instructed fire to put itself together as the sun above, and earth got orders
to collect itself as the soil below. Both fire and earth felt an agreeable sense of
purpose once they were fitting in to the new scheme of things, and it wasn't
long before metal and water joined in, too.

Having created space and direction, the tree at the center of the universe
began to grow. As it grew, it needed raw materials to make wood. It used what
was at hand: fire, earth, metal and water. These were organized into something
new and unique: an individual self made of the elements, but somehow separate from them. This was the first protagonist.

As it continued to grow, the protagonist-tree got older. That is to say, it moved into the future. Until now there had been no future to move into. With no growth and no development, nothing had ever happened, or at least nothing that would contrast with anything else. Each moment was indistinguishable from every other, and time was non-existent. But the growth of the tree put an end to that. Now there was direction in time as well as in space, and the tree began to look ahead and plan how it would proceed with its growth. So the tree became the first visionary and to its pioneering efforts we are indebted for our ability to see. But we are getting ahead of our proto-story.

As the tree was growing and looking into the future, it foresaw the problem of death and for that problem it came up with a fun solution: sex. Of course, sex requires the presence of another individual, so the tree asked Dreamer to dream up an appealing mate. In a trice, a second tree appeared near by. The first tree became desperately infatuated and wanted to start reproducing immediately. The second tree had its own plans, though. It was more interested in branching out on its own personal growth before putting down roots and raising seedlings. Inevitably, the two quarreled and the new tree stalked off. If it hadn't changed its mind the universe would still be paralyzed with anger, but thankfully, the two got together and started a family.

So it was that Dreamer put a tree at the center of the universe and from that tree were born time, space, individuality, conflict, sex and death. Of course it is no coincidence that these are the ingredients of a good yarn and the first one the tree spun is still one of the best: boy meets girl, boy loses girl, boy gets girl back. Since then, every time a seedling sprouts, dozens of new stories sprout with it, so Dreamer hasn't been bored for a moment.

It is springtime. A willow seed sprouts and starts growing up to be a tree. It will never be a blade of grass. Never a trout or a termite. It will become a willow tree. It has the inner vision of willowness and will consult this vision like a blueprint at every occasion. "Hmm, let's see.... We have good sunshine. Water supplies, minerals, and soil nutrients are holding up, so yes, there is an opportunity for further expansion. Shall we add some fins? Let's check the plan.... No, no, not fins; we're supposed to be putting on wood. Willow wood at that." Now the willow has to decide exactly how and where it will put the wood. Shall it grow low and bushy or tall and slender? Shall it grow straight, or shall it lean a bit this way or that to get more light? Which of its branches shall grow first? Maybe they should all grow at the same time? There are thousands of decisions to be made.

I am not much different from a willow. I, too, am growing, consulting the vision I carry in my soul, and making decisions about how to make that vision into reality. There is this difference between the way willow grows and the way I do: willow's body keeps getting taller until her last day, whereas I achieved my full height thirty-three years ago. Whatever growth I have achieved since then has been in my mind and spirit. I have a lot of growing to do in these areas, because my education stunted me.

My experiences in school were not exceptionally traumatic; in fact, I was a "successful" student. I say my education stunted me not because of what I had, but because of what I didn't have: initiation. Initiation is a ritual that shows a person his or her purpose in life. In traditional societies this ritual is usually performed near the time of puberty, because it marks the moment when physical growth is complete and education of the soul can begin. The perception of life purpose is the dawn of spiritual vision; before this, the soul is wandering in the dark, so initiation is also often called the "vision quest." There are many ways of performing the ritual, but it is always done under the guidance of elders. Often initiates are isolated from their families and undergo fasting and other hardships in the wilderness. Eventually they are visited by spirits who show them their life path and grant spiritual powers to help them along. The initiates return to society knowing how to contribute to their people. They are now young adults growing up to be elders themselves.[1]

Despite the fact that I went through the outer form of initiation when I had my bar mitzvah, as a young man I was utterly ignorant. It didn't matter that I had a lot of formal education; without vision I knew nothing I needed to know. When I was in my twenties, my father often asked me when I was going to stop floundering. It made me furious to hear him say that. I maintained that I wasn't floundering, but he was right; I was floundering. Part of my fury was having to admit it. The other part was natural anger that no one had helped me find my direction. The closest I got was taking a vocational aptitude test from a guidance counselor in high school. The results showed that I could be successful at any work I chose with the exception of agriculture and medicine.

My initiation was late, slow and informal—a series of vision quests and other experiences that stretched over more than a decade starting after I turned thirty. At that I was fortunate. Many people today never find out what their purpose in life is. They have no way to express their

---

1. Since initiation is a growth process powered by the Wood element, it is fascinating to note that the first instructor on a vision quest is often a tree spirit. Two recent accounts of this phenomenon come to mind: the initiation of Ron Geyshick, a Lac La Croix Ojibway healer (See Te Bwe Win Summerhill Press, Toronto 1989), and that of Malidoma Somé, a Dagara shaman from West Africa (*Ritual: Power, Healing and Community*, Swan•Raven & Co., Newberg, OR 1993).

creative power, and so each day is as monotonous and frustrating as the last.

Modern life opens a path not to the soul but to the shopping mall, and the force of growth has been diverted onto this path. The result is economic growth—the rapid conversion of nature into toxic junk. This is what we call the "gross national product," and unless it gets a bit grosser every year, our "economy" founders. There is a word for out-of-control rapid growth: cancer. Cancer continues to spread in our bodies and on the earth because, like trees, we must have growth. The only way out is to rediscover that material growth is a youthful phase that prepares the way for real growth into elderhood.

In the short run, the prospects for rediscovery do not look good. The mass media show that we worship youth and want to prolong it as long as possible. The cruelty of this cult cuts deeper than the plastic surgeon's knife. Our culture throws elders on the scrap heap as soon as their prime consumer years are over.

I am not the only person angry about being kept in the dark. Deep down most people resent the assumption that they were born to shop. This resentment is healthy, for anger provides power to overcome obstacles. The anger that drives people to meaningless jobs could also destroy the whole frustrating economic system. An explosive change of this type is unlikely, though, because our frustration is enfeebled by denial and alcohol.

When George Bush visited Russia as President of the United States, newspapers in this country carried front-page photos of him hoisting glasses of vodka with President Gorbachev. Would it be conceivable that the two heads of state could publicly toast each other with a dangerous drug other than alcohol? Cocaine maybe, or heroin?

When the Spaniards arrived in Mexico five hundred years ago, they encountered a civilization much more advanced than their own. This civilization prized pulque, or agave wine, but inebriation was severely punishable by law for any but the elderly. After destroying this civilization and subjecting its people to slavery, the Europeans introduced a long list of new restrictive laws. However, the invaders made distilled spirits available for the first time and removed any legal sanction against drunkenness.

In order to understand the privileged place of alcohol we must note that the liver is the seat of the Wood. The liver harbors the spiritual soul and is the source of vision, growth and creativity. It is also the seat of anger. The Plan for our life is to be found here. Alcohol devastates the liver. Years before cirrhosis sets in, the vision of the soul is lost. The alcoholic forgets what he or she is angry about. This may partially explain the epidemic of alcoholism among Native Americans. People who have been raped, beaten, robbed, massacred and abused in every conceivable way are now taking out their rage on their own bodies and those of their spouses and children. But angry drunks are no problem compared to sober people who might remember the reasons for their anger. Thanks to alcohol, business goes on as usual at the mall.

Whatever your cultural heritage, if no one showed you your life's purpose, your spiritual development was neglected. It doesn't matter where your ancestors were born; the economic juggernaut packs the booze wherever it goes. You live in a nation of alcoholics. And business goes on as usual at the mall.

However snarled and hopeless the human dream gets, though, wild plants still willingly take people into their paradise. I don't know how they do that. It is a mystery I love to ponder and probably will never solve, which is fine with me because I like mysteries. I just keep asking the plants for their magic and admiring it when it comes.

Edna's life was certainly snarled and hopeless when one of my colleagues brought her to see me. She said she had chronic fatigue syndrome, by which she meant that she had done very little but lie in bed for two years. The feeling she had was as if a giant were pinning her to the ground, making it impossible to move. This was her way of saying her Wood was thwarted and unable to grow, and the green tinge on her face, the shouting tone of her voice, her angry demeanor, and the rancid odor of her body confirmed this evaluation. After pointing this out to Donna Guillemin, my colleague and former student, I left Edna in her care.

When I saw Edna again six months later she was all smiles. "I've got some wild stories to tell you, Eliot," she said.

"Tell me," I said.

"Well, for one thing, you know I used to be violently allergic," Edna began.

"No, I don't think you told me that," I interrupted.

"Well, yes, I was. But after a few sessions with Donna, I noticed an amazing improvement. I said, 'Donna, what have you been giving me, anyway?' and she said that it was scotch broom. 'Scotch broom?' I said, 'That stuff used to be my nemesis.' A while back I went into a restaurant and got a horrible asthma attack. I looked around but I couldn't see anything that would be setting it off, so I asked the waiter if there was any scotch broom around. He pointed way over to the other side of this huge room. There on the mantle was a tiny dried sprig of it. He said it had been there for years. I couldn't breathe well enough to eat my meal, so I left, and the asthma went away almost immediately. When I told this story to Donna I mentioned that since she started treating me, broom and I have become friends! And I went and stuck my face right into a big scotch broom bush in full flower just to prove it! No ill effects whatsoever!

"Here's another thing," Edna continued, sticking her outstretched fingers in front of my face. Her fingernails were long, strong and healthy-looking. Previously they had been yellow, rotting and disfigured with fungus growth. This was a significant sign, for according to Chinese physiology the health of the nails depends on the health of the liver.

"That's fantastic, Edna," I said. "But what about your fatigue?"

"Oh, that," she said. "No, I haven't been tired anymore. In fact, for the first time I feel like I know what I'm supposed to be doing with my life, and I've gone back to school to start preparing for a new career."

QUESTIONS: WOOD AND YOU

These questions can help you see how you grow. Stand with your back against a tall tree. Imagine that your spine is the trunk and your head is above the treetops. From this vantage point you can see the landscape of your whole life. Answer the questions clearly and truthfully.

1. How do you feel in spring?
2. What are your pet peeves?
3. When has it been difficult for you to make a decision?
4. How do you feel when your plans are thwarted?
5. When was the last time you shouted at someone?
6. When was the last time you wanted to shout at someone?
7. How do you feel in green clothes? In a green room?
8. Do you have a green thumb?
9. Is your closet organized? Your pockets? Purse? Desk?
10. Do you enjoy organizing people and events?
11. How coordinated are you?
12. How is your vision?
13. How are your fingernails and toenails?
14. How often do you drink alcohol? Why?
15. What frustrates you?

16. How do you feel in windy weather?
17. Do you enjoy sour, acid foods?
18. Have you ever been angry enough to cry?
19. How is your sense of direction? How are you at giving directions?
20. Did you have any developmental problems as a child?
21. What were the circumstances of your birth?
22. What are your experiences and feelings about childbirth?
23. How would you like your life to be five years from now? Ten years from now?
24. Do you have plans for your old age?
25. What creative activities do you enjoy? How often?
26. What new ideas or concepts have you come up with?
27. How are you a better person today than ten years ago?
28. What are your dreams in life? Your hopes for the future?
29. When have you felt full of hope?
30. What is the purpose of your life?

As you answer the questions, notice how responsive you are to the process of growth in your life at this moment. Like trees, we grow in different seasons and in different soils. What season of growth are you in right now? How fast or slow is it? What type of growth is it? What are the obstacles to your growth? As you cycle through different stages of growth through out your life, how is the one you are in now similar to some other period in your life? Refocus on the tree you've been with. Ask this great teacher what you need to do to open your life more to growth and change within you. Visualize roots going down into the earth from your body next to this tree and then mentally draw leaves sprouting and blossoms and fruits coming forth from you. Rejoice that you are growing. Feel the frustration of the places in you where you are being thwarted. Touch the upward thrust of your life: Wood.

Blocks to Treatment

Possession

Conventional medical care ends at death, and this is a blessing for many who spend their last days in the hospital. On the other hand, shamans know that sometimes the soul is confused after death and cannot find its way to the next world without help. In fact, with sudden violent death or suicide, the departed person is often unaware of having left his or her body. The soul may wander about confounded by its inability to get what it wants. Coming across someone whose defenses are weak, the dead may enter "holes" or gaps in that person's soul. Once inside, the dead person manipulates the life of the live one. This is the most common form of possession.

As our people become weaker in spirit, and as we neglect our dead, possession becomes more common. In nineteen years of practice, I have noticed a huge rise in the number of possessed people I see. We can't do anything about this epidemic until we acknowledge its existence, and so far we are taking the attitude that possession is superstitious nonsense or Hollywood sensationalism. In exploiting our fears about this, authors and filmmakers draw attention from the fact that possession does not usually result in bizarre behavior. In our country there are hundreds of thousands of possessed people living normal middle-class lives. These are not members of satanic cults; they are perfectly nice people. Their problem is that the lives they are living are not their own because their souls are out of reach. When you look into their eyes, you see nothing more than their pupils.

I suspected my patient Janice might be suffering from possession, so I made a dream journey to find out for sure. I was led to some broad stone steps in front of a Spanish mission in Tucson, Arizona. There were a number of Native Americans chatting and selling their wares on the steps. Judging from their dress I guessed the time was about 200 years ago. My attention was drawn in particular to one young mother who was playing with her four-year-old daughter. The little girl was wearing striking red moccasins. Suddenly the militia appeared. Without warning or provocation they opened fire on the Indians, and the little girl with the red moccasins died in her mother's arms. The mother raised her head to see her attackers. In that moment she too was struck by a musket ball. She died instantly, with no physical pain, and so was unaware of her death. Her soul remained on the steps searching for her beloved little girl.

Two hundred years later, Janice, a sensitive, traumatized four-year-old girl in a pair of red shoes, came to play on the mission stairs. The Indian woman attached herself to her with all the passion in her embittered heart and stayed with her for thirty years. The little girl Janice was now a grown woman, but was still living the Indian woman's pain.

In the dream journey, I approached the woman. She looked at me suspiciously. "What do you want?" she asked me.

"I noticed you were unhappy, so I came to help," I said. "I know you want to be with your daughter. I can take you to see her."

"What are you talking about?" she snarled. "My daughter is right here." She motioned toward Janice.

"Pardon me, but there must be some mistake," I countered. "This is a white person. You are an Indian. She cannot possibly be your daughter. Have a look for yourself. Put your arm next to hers. See the difference in color."

She compared skin colors. What she saw left her speechless. I went on. "I think you must have got confused somehow. You see, this is a woman of your own age. Your daughter is only about four years old. Isn't that so?" She nodded and then burst into tears. I stepped to her side and put my hand on her shoulder comfortingly. "Your daughter is in a faraway land, a different world. She is very eager to see you. She has been waiting for you for a long time. I can take you to her. Will you come with me?" She nodded her assent.

I had no idea how to find the little girl who had died so many years ago, but I was confident my spirit helpers would know. I took the mother by the hand and asked to be lead. We were taken to a heavenly realm like those depicted in certain religious paintings. Shafts of golden light descended between fluffy clouds, and choirs of angels sang to greet us. I left daughter and mother in a tearful, happy embrace, and returned to my office.

"Janice," I asked, "where did you grow up?"

"In Tucson," she replied.

"Aha. And is there a Spanish mission in Tucson?"

"There sure is. I used to go to mass there. In front of the church there are some broad stone steps that I used to play on. That was my favorite place in the whole world. It's kind of strange, really, because when I got older I found out that a terrible massacre happened on those steps. About two hundred years ago, the army killed a whole bunch of Indians in cold blood there. It gives me the creeps to think about it."

"Amazing!" I said. "Tell me something else, Janice. When you were about four, did you happen to have a pair of red shoes?"

"How did you know that?" she said.

Although possession is usually caused without any malicious intent, a person skilled in such things can deliberately induce it.

"There was this woman who was working with me at the television station," Rosilyn said. "We joked and kidded around, but we were competing with each other underneath. She used to tell me that she was into black magic. She would brag about how she had got the best of different people by putting curses on them. I didn't pay any attention because I didn't believe in that stuff. Anyway, after a while, she started pulling these maneuvers to get me out of the program I was working on. We had an argument, and later I said something that got her in trouble with the station manager. A couple of days later she came by my desk and sprinkled water all over me. 'You don't have to do that, I've already had a shower this morning,' I told her. I was sarcastic. I didn't take it seriously. But from that moment on my life has been going downhill. I couldn't get any decent assignments any more. I started to feel terribly insecure. My energy declined. And at night I started to sense an evil presence around me, like someone wanting to rape me."

Rather than dealing with Rosilyn's co-worker or the spirit she summoned, I called upon what traditional Chinese doctors call "The Seven Dragons for Seven Demons." In Oriental mythology, the dragon is an auspicious bringer of divine power and blessing, and within every human being there are seven dragon spirits who can consume possessing entities. I asked one of my plant spirit allies to rouse Rosilyn's dragons. The demon was dispatched quickly, and Rosilyn's life turned in the right direction.

Soul Loss

A person who is strong and whole need not fear possession. It can only happen when an entity finds a gap in the soul of a weakened host. Most of us realize trauma can make us weak, but many do not know we can lose part of our soul. When we confront pain too great to bear, part of our soul may leave and inhabit a different dream. This response enables us to survive trauma, but if the part that left never comes back, we are left less than whole. Even if we don't get possessed, we may not have enough soul force to ward off disease, depression, fatigue and disaster. The remedy for this is for someone to search the dream worlds to retrieve the missing pieces.

My spirits taught me to bring back soul pieces for others, and I practiced it occasionally for several years. When Sandra Ingerman came out with *Soul Retrieval*, her excellent book on the subject, more people became interested in this kind of healing and I started doing it more often. My experience with Debra convinced me to do this work as a matter of routine.

Debra had been under the care of some of the finest acupuncturists in the world for several years and then had come to me for plant spirit medicine. She had made improvements in her health, but much remained unresolved. One day I got a phone call from a mutual friend telling me that Debra had undergone emergency surgery for blockage of the intestine and was in the hospital in a distant city. Two weeks later the same friend called again to say that Debra had been transferred to a local hospital. Although the operation had been successful, she had not recovered, and medical tests had failed to determine what was keeping her from getting well.

After work I drove to the hospital to visit Debra. I found her shockingly thin and frail. Her voice was feeble and her arms and hands hung limp on the bed as she spoke. The presence of death hung in the air around her bed. I summoned a plant spirit for her. Her pulse responded, but the presence still hovered.

I then made a dream journey to her soul, and what her soul chose to show me was a vivid scene of sexual abuse at the age of four in which her father was the perpetrator. The four-year-old said, "I can't take this any more," and then left this world, soaring towards a land of comfort in an orange sun. It took a lot of coaxing and cajoling on my part to convince that four-year-old soul to return to her adult life, but finally she agreed and I brought her back to Debra's body.

Returning to ordinary reality, I found Debra more alert. The death pall was gone.

"I had a vision while you were doing whatever you were doing," she told me.

"Tell me about it," I said.

"Someone gave me a little girl. I got up and walked to the front door of the hospital. It was a huge heavy oak door with a bar across it, but I just smashed through it and walked out of this place with that little girl in my arms."

"That's wonderful, Debra! And you look better already! But listen, I'd like you to tell me a little more about what's been happening to you. Why did you leave town? What where you doing just before you got sent to the hospital?"

"I went to see my therapist," she said. "This woman is working with my inner child. That morning we had a big breakthrough. For the first time I was able to recover memories of sexual abuse by my father when I was four years old. It was very heavy. I guess I couldn't deal with it, because that afternoon I went to the emergency room with pain in the abdomen, and they operated right away.

"It is strange; I have memories of what was happening to my soul while I was under anesthesia. A woman came and held out her hands to me. It was very comforting, very safe. She told me that if I just took her hands, I wouldn't have to come back to this world. I didn't take her hands, but I didn't really decide to come back either. It's as if some part of me has been trying to make up its mind. The doctors are puzzled; they can't figure out why I haven't been getting better, but I know the reason."

Evidently, restoring her lost soul part was what she needed to bring her back to life, because the next morning Debra got out of bed, packed her suitcase, and checked herself out of the hospital. She went straight home, phoned her father and confronted him with her experience. The father, a psychiatrist, denied any wrongdoing, and tried to convince Debra that she was insane. He was taking the next airplane to her city to have her committed to a mental institution, he warned. And he had a key to her apartment.

Debra packed her suitcase for a second time. When her father arrived, she and her fiancé were safely out of town.

Husband/Wife Imbalance

In addition to possession and soul loss, there is a third disease factor unknown to modern medicine. This factor in a way is more serious than the other two, because if unaddressed, it eventually causes premature death. This cause of disease is called the "husband/wife imbalance."

To understand husband/wife imbalance, we can start by coming to terms with husband/wife *balance*. Everyone needs both masculine and feminine qualities to survive in this world. We need a bit of the active, aggressive, go-getter, and we also need some of the nurturing, supportive, let-it-be attitude. These two should support each other, like the husband and wife in a caveman marriage. The husband is endowed by nature to be a hunter: he has the muscle and the temperament to kill.

The wife is endowed by nature to care for the family: she has the breasts and the temperament to feed the young.

As long as husband and wife fulfill their respective duties, the family survives. But imagine what would happen if one day the husband comes home, flops himself down on a hide, and says to his wife, "Honey, I'm sick and tired of this rat race. All I do is chase mammoths. No sooner do I drag one home than you guys devour it and then I have to go out and find another one. I've had it! From now on I'm going to stay around the fire and take it easy like you. You go out and bring home the meat!" No doubt the wife would do quite well out hunting with the boys, but what would happen to the young ones at home? With no breast to turn to, they would soon starve to death. If this went on long enough, the family would die out.

If the wife suddenly announced she was sick of being oppressed, sick of staying around the camp, and from now on she was darn well going to insist on her right to have fun killing animals like her husband, of course the result would be the same.

Before I make myself persona non grata with the women's movement and the men's movement alike, remember that I insist everyone, whether man or woman, has both the husband and the wife energies within. We all have to be part hunter, part nurturer.

Imbalance between the husband and the wife brings death. It could be by disease, suicide, or accident, but it is always an unnatural, unhappy death. Often a person who is suffering from husband/wife imbalance will sense that death is near long before there is any medical reason to think so. As the masculine, aggressive principle weakens and resigns itself, the person loses vitality. Glenda, a sixty-year old housewife, came to me in this condition. Her fatigue was so great she could barely move. Medical doctors had found that an antibody was destroying her thyroid hormone as fast as it could be formed, but they were unable to correct the problem. A host of non-conventional therapists had no success either. As she climbed onto my treatment couch, Glenda confessed in a whisper that she felt she was not long for this world, but as soon as my plant friends got husband and wife to stop fighting over the thyroid secretions, she was full of vitality again.

Bob was an airline pilot who complained, "Nothing seems to matter to me anymore. Life doesn't interest me. When I'm not working, I just lie around all the time. This isn't like me. I've always been a happy, highly motivated kind of guy. I enjoyed work, and I enjoyed working on projects at home when I wasn't flying.

"I have some physical complaints, too," Bob continued. "I'm eating huge amounts of food. I'm hungry all the time, but I just don't seem to get the value out of what I'm eating. Also, my wife and I have been trying to have a baby, but no luck. The doctors checked us both out...she's okay, but my sperm count is just about nonexistent. This worries me a lot, and yet sometimes I think maybe it's for the best that we haven't had a baby, because ever since I haven't been feeling well, I can't tolerate my wife. She can say just the simplest little thing, and it throws me into a blind rage. I can't control myself."

Bob's symptoms dramatized the state of the broken inner marriage. The husband within was henpecked, impotent and enraged at his inner wife, who was letting her husband go hungry.

It is interesting to note that no amount of conventional medical treatment and no amount of marital counseling would have helped Bob's foundering inner marriage. Correcting the inner husband/wife imbalance had dramatic results, though. He came back five days after the treatment and I recorded his words verbatim:

> The change in me is indescribable! The moment I walked out of here last time, I burst into laughter! I couldn't stop laughing! What a relief! I've finally come back to life. I've got my energy back and I've been working around the house again. I haven't noticed the hunger so much, and I haven't lost my temper with my wife.

Within six weeks Bob had his sperm count taken again. It was more than four times what it was before the plant spirits brought his husband and wife together again.

Remedies

Gil Milner is a distinguished physician with an impressive list of credentials. Among other things, he is a neurologist, a psychiatrist, a child psychiatrist and a former Professor of Medicine at a major university. Several years ago, he attended one of my trainings. I couldn't help but wonder how a person with his background would relate to the spirits of plants, so after each dream journey I peeked over his shoulder to see what he was writing in his notebook. In each case, I saw esoteric-looking squiggles with syllables jotted below them in a foreign language.

After several days, my curiosity overcame my embarrassment about peeking. "What is that strange stuff you write in your notebook, Gil?" I asked.

"Oh, you know, it's the song of the plant," he answered.

"How's that?"

"Well, each plant gives you its power in the form of a song, right?"

"I don't know. Does it?" I asked.

"Sure! Don't they sing to you?"

"No. They haven't yet."

"Hmm, I thought they did that with everybody. Look, this is a kind of notation to remember the melody, and these are the words of the song written underneath," said Dr. Milner, showing me his notebook.

On the final day of the course, after the students had treated each other, I approached him. "Everyone has been treated now except me," I said. "I would like to ask you for a treatment."

"Yes, of course. I would be happy to treat you," he replied.

I said, "Forget about pills and tinctures, though. I want you to sing me my medicine."

The doctor blushed, looked at his feet, and stammered something incoherent. Looking up again he saw I was determined, so he nodded and I lay down on the treatment table so he could interview me and take my pulses. After that procedure he disappeared into the next room with the other students to discuss what plant should be sung. A few minutes later they reappeared. He picked up my drum and played a slow loping rhythm and then began to sing a repetitive, strangely beautiful chant. It was absolutely authoritative. I felt the song enter my chest. Tears came to my eyes. Dr. Milner picked up the tempo and lifted my mood; I smiled. He stopped singing and checked my pulses and then all the students once again went into the next room to consult.

When they returned he drummed and chanted as before, but this time the effect was deeper, more internal. I closed my eyes and suddenly lost consciousness of everything that was happening in the room. I found myself in the woods, sitting on a forest floor that was carpeted with wild ginger. The song of the ginger was pouring out of the mouths of its purple flowers, offering me treasures: heart-shaped leaves, rich soil, breezes sighing in the graceful arms of maples, and certain other wordless blessings.

Gil stopped singing and I returned to the classroom. "Wild ginger," I said. "Asarum canadense." He nodded and checked my pulse, even though he already must have known that a splendid treatment had been done. I got up and gave him a hug to express my thanks. His face was red, his eyes full of tears, and he trembled noticeably. "How are you doing?" I asked.

"Wherever I travel," he said, "the shamans always seek me out. They give me their feathers. I've got a whole drawer full of them at home. I could never figure out why they do that. 'I'm a doctor,' I would say to myself. 'I'm not going to use their kind of medicine.' But now I know why."

Plant spirit medicine is a magico-religious rite in which plant gods bestow their grace. How is that grace invoked? Some people use song, others use pills and potions, still others lay on hands, wave feathers, or dance. Who knows how many ways may be waiting to be discovered or rediscovered?

Whatever method is used, the spirits are invited to help the patient enter the dream of nature; this has nothing to do with fighting illness. For us, there is no such thing as an herb that is good for arthritis or migraine or depression or cancer. Whatever medicine a plant spirit gives you, that's what it will do for your patients. As the Matses Indians in the Amazon told Peter Gorman, if you want to use a plant for healing, you have to dream it or it won't work for you. Rarely do two people have exactly the same dreams. Rarely do two people use the same plant in exactly the same way.

Even conventional herbalists will privately admit that their art is highly personal. The successes of one herbalist cannot be duplicated by another using the same remedies. There are two standardized herbal systems that are notable exceptions to this: medical herbalism and homeopathy.

Medical herbalism is currently enjoying a renewal of popularity in Japan and Germany where scientific research and clinical trials are being done with herbal compounds. Although this method is preferable to the development of synthetic drugs, the analytical double-blind approach excludes the possibility of healing the mind or spirit. (See chapter four.)

Homeopathy is a healing method that employs rigorous empirical methods to discover which symptoms a given medicine will provoke. Samuel Hahnemann, the founder of homeopathy, considered plants to be morbific agents given to bring on an artificial disease similar to the natural one the patient suffers from. This stimulates the patient's recuperative powers to overcome both diseases very quickly. While homeopathy is highly effective when skillfully applied, it relates to plants and healing in an utterly different way from plant spirit medicine. Conscientious homeopathic doctors follow Samuel Hahnemann, while plant spirit medicine practitioners enter the dream of nature on their own.

The Bach Flower Remedies are an outgrowth of homeopathy. Dr. Bach, an English homeopathic physician, was sensitive to the power of plants to heal negative emotional states. He set out to create a simple system of medicine that could be practiced by anyone without special training, and he succeeded at his goal. To do so, he had to sacrifice depth and power in the name of easy application. In the Bach Flowers, a plant essence is given to dispel a corresponding negative emotion. No effort is made to diagnose or treat the underlying cause of the emotion. By contrast, from the point of view of plant spirit medicine a given emotional problem might be caused by a number of factors such as an imbalance of one of the elements, possession, or husband/wife imbalance. It takes years of work to acquire the skills needed to detect and root out these factors.

I believe it is unfair and unreasonable to expect an unskilled person to unlock the greatest healing power of plants. This is especially true when someone attempts to heal himself or herself. Self-healing does sometimes occur, of course, but it is the exception rather than the rule because illness usually takes root in our emotional blind spot. Disease is a call for help, and often the best way to help ourselves is to take the help of others. Exaggerated independence is one of the attitudes that isolates us and makes us ill. Healing can be a celebration of our connectedness and interdependence.

Michael Harner tells an anecdote about an Indian shaman he met in the Amazon during the 1950s. Harner was impressed by the young man's power and also enjoyed his company, and the two became friends. Before Michael's to return to the United States, he invited his friend to make shamanic dream journeys to Berkeley so they could continue their friendship. Much to Michael's surprise the powerful shaman appeared crestfallen. "I cannot do this," he said. "Why not?" Michael asked. "I've seen you do much greater things!" The Indian replied, "I cannot visit you in Berkeley because I do not know the trails." This was his way of saying there is no substitute for experience.

The same thing holds true for someone who wants to learn the medicine of plants: there is no substitute for experience. This medicine comes from intimacy with living plants. Just as no one would think of trying to make babies with a character in a novel, no one should think of trying to make medicine with a plant in a book—not even this book. I will describe some of my intimacies, but yours would be different.

One of my favorite plants for helping with Fire imbalance is scarlet pimpernel, *anagallis arvensis*. This is a familiar wayside plant in America, Europe and other parts of the world. It is a low, sprawling herb with tiny flowers that are usually salmon-colored with a magenta center and bright yellow stamens. They open in sunny weather and close tight when it is dark or cloudy. The taste of this herb is bitter and offensive and is said to be somewhat poisonous. All in all, this is a difficult plant to get intimate with, but well worth the effort. In English herbalism it had a reputation for dispelling melancholy, and Somerset folk still know it as "Laughter Bringer."

My dream journey to the spirit of this plant took me through long stretches of cold dark space until I arrived at a small distant planet. The sphere seemed deserted until I got to the remotest part, where I saw a gruff unshaven man dressed in a tight t-shirt and black pants.

"Are you the spirit of scarlet pimpernel?" I asked.

"What's it to ya?"

"Well, I...."

"Listen, buddy, why don't you just take off to the next solar system. There's some nice flowers over there. Scram."

This had to be the spirit of scarlet pimpernel! He was showing the same bitterness and the same over-protectiveness in the dream as he did in waking reality. I remembered that the warmth of the sun would get him to open up and share his beauty.

"I love your flowers!" I said. "They have the wildest color combination! It makes me happy to look at them! You must be a beautiful guy behind that gruff front!" He cracked a little smile and blushed. I went on, "What are you doing here all alone on this frigid little planet?"

A tear trickled down the tough guy's cheek. "People are so cold, so heartless!" he said. "They can hurt you if you let your guard down. I take everything to heart—I'm just too vulnerable, I guess."

He didn't need to say any more to let me know he had medicine for the heart protector. When he saw I understood his act, he threw back his head and laughed uninhibitedly. "May I use you?" I asked. "Will you share your medicine with others?" In reply he took my hands and we danced in a circle, abandoning ourselves to joy.

Mullein, *verbascum thapsus,* is another herb common in both the New World and the Old. The leaves are soft, fuzzy and flannel-like. Second-year plants put up a tall central stalk tipped with bright yellow sweet-smelling flowers. A warm infusion of these flowers in olive oil is used as eardrops for children's earaches.

Often in my dreams of plants, I see nothing and hear nothing, yet experience a definite inner sensation. If the sensation is disagreeable, I assume the plant can heal it; if it is agreeable, I assume the plant spirit is showing me the benefits it has to offer. My dream with mullein was this way. Nothing "happened," yet I felt coddled and secure as if my mother had just given me warm milk, tucked me into bed with mullein-flannel sheets, and sung me a sweet lullaby. Since that time, I have used mullein to bring comfort and security to many people who suffered from imbalance of the Earth.

Plantain *(plantago ssp.)* is a native of Europe that has accompanied the European peoples in the colonization of the world. Some Native American tribes referred to this plant as "white man's footsteps," because it was found wherever the newcomers trod. It is a soft, bland plant whose young leaves can be eaten as salad. This softness is balanced by tremendous strength; plantain competes well among the toughest grasses. In fact, if you live in a temperate climate, you probably have plantain growing in your lawn or the nearest park.

Plantago psyllium is the source of psyllium seeds, which constitute the main ingredient in many commercial bulk laxatives. Plantain has many other uses as well among folk herbalists. It has been a favorite of mine since my farm days in Vermont because the juice when introduced into a suppurating lesion will eliminate most of the infection and inflammation within twenty-four hours.

As I already mentioned, plantain was the first plant I dreamed with. The spirit appeared to me as a winged fairy holding a magic wand in one hand and a vial of sleeping potion in the other. I could use her medicine, she said, for the mental and spiritual equivalents of pus and constipation. She called herself a gentle but powerful purifier of the soul. She let me know she could bring purity and sparkle where old filth had polluted the mind; thus her strongest affinity is to the Metal element and the colon in particular. When such problems cause insomnia, her medicine is doubly indicated.

The stream orchids of Western North America and the helleborine orchids of Eastern North America and Europe all belong to the genus *epipactis* and all have similar medicine. Visiting the live plant, I enjoyed the complex beauty of the flowers, but I was even more struck with an unusual sensation I felt when grasping the leaf. It was as if the plant were holding my hand in a reassuring way. This is what I wrote in my notebook after my dream with *epipactis gigantea:*

> This is a very companionable spirit, like an old and trusted friend. There is no need to speak with it, for we understand each other so well. Telepathically it told me that this is an elixir for loneliness, fear and agitation coming from the Water element. Its effect is a deep calming presence, like viewing a still pond in tranquillity with my life's companion by my side. This spirit is completely loyal, a reliable aid for separation anxiety.
>
> Its action comes from its willingness to share the peace of its home. The plant is made of the vibrations that surround it. Observe well the home it selects: moist, shady, undisturbed. It only grows in magical places, feeding on peace and storing it in its flesh.

Throughout the world, pussy willow is the messenger of spring, foretelling the rebirth of nature. Willows *(salix ssp.)* make medicine for the Wood. Indeed, these trees offer a wonderful example of the qualities of Wood in balance. Anyone who has worked with willow knows that it bends where other woods break. On the other hand, the sheer strength of the growth force in the willow is unsurpassed. A dry stick inserted into moist soil will sprout roots and leaves.

To those whose Wood has become rigid and who are frustrated, uptight or clumsy, willow brings grace and flexibility. To the drifters, the hopeless and the stunted whose Wood has become feeble, the willow spirit brings a surge of power, a vision of the future, and new growth.

The Chinese written word for "acupuncture" consists of two characters: the first depicts a needle piercing the skin and the second represents the fluffy dried leaves of mugwort, *artemisia vulgaris*. Mugwort is indispensable to the acupuncturist's art because the energy of the plant is virtually identical to the energy in the human body. Small cones of dried mugwort are burned at acupuncture points on the body to stimulate the patient's vitality.

Mugwort is highly regarded wherever it is found. Among some California Native Americans, it is a sacred plant of divination and spiritual healing. It is important in Mesoamerican folk medicine. In certain European traditions, sprigs of the herb are placed under the pillow to provoke vivid dreams, and the plant has been linked with the practice of magic since Anglo-Saxon times.

In plant spirit medicine, mugwort also occupies a prominent position, for it is the most important of the remedies that are used to effect transfers of energy within the meridian system. These transfers are called for in many instances. For example, sometimes energy can get blocked as it flows from one meridian to the next. It can also happen that the energy in one side of the body becomes markedly less than the energy on the other side, causing lopsided functioning. Both problems can be detected through skillful reading of the Chinese pulses, and both are remedied by the mugwort spirit.

Mugwort is an acknowledged expert at moving energy, and since matter is but a dense form of energy, this herb can actually be used to correct structural problems of the body. Mugwort structural work offers an alternative to chiropractic or osteopathic adjustments, and preliminary experiments with Hellerwork (an offshoot of Rolfing) show that it also has great potential in soft-tissue bodywork.

Another category of plant spirit medicines are those that bring something special to the mind and spirit without having any particular elemental correspondence. There is a varied range of effects available from these remedies. I will mention just two of my favorites: wood anemone and St. Johnswort.

Here is a transcription of my initial field notes on wood anemone (*anemone lyallii* in the West, *anemone quinquefolia* in the East, and *anemone nemorosa* in Europe):

A slender nymph or gnome appeared and flew silently away. I followed. We landed on a rock ledge and waited quietly for the right moment. It led me through a narrow cleft. Inside there was a cave which opened into a large room with a stone idol in the center. The idol came to life and got on its hands and knees, giving me a ride on its back. It turned into a turtle and walked serenely to the river. We plunged in and stayed on the bottom.

An enigmatic journey, but I think the point is this: The problems and cares of life loom like the cedars and firs of the forest where the lowly anemone lives. Entering the world of the plant spirits requires lightness, quickness, and timing—to slip unnoticed through the cracks of the rock, or ordinary waking state. So anemone is to be used before another remedy, particularly when the patient is dense or preoccupied with worldly problems. This will lead the second remedy into the patient's cave (skull) and introduce it to the stone idol (god of his consciousness). Then the two can play together at the bottom of the stream (of awareness).

St. Johnswort (hypericum perforatum) is a perennial favorite of herbalists and plant magicians. Every age and system has found a use for this herb. It was a vulnerary for Christian forces during the Crusades. A recent vogue in European herbalism as an anti-depressant replaces its earlier fame as an exorcist. In homeopathy, it is the sine qua non for nerve damage of all kinds. Only in the American West, where it is known as "Klamath weed," is it not revered; on the contrary it has been the target of chemical eradication campaigns because it invades pasture and range land.

My dream of St. Johnswort was short and simple. A disembodied voice told me, "I will bind together that which has been rent asunder." Since that time, I have used it as cement for fractured souls. It works wonders in cases of soul loss, husband/wife imbalance, possession and other situations such as the following:

A woman in her early twenties consulted me with complaints of severe fatigue that had started several months previously. She was active and energetic before then. In questioning her, I discovered that in the nine months before the onset of her illness she had two abortions. Her boyfriend was very supportive, she said, and they both agreed this was the best thing to do. She said she loved her boyfriend and they planned to have children later. Her voice sounded quite even as she reported that she had no issues with the abortions. But this was just her mind reporting. Her spirit was saying that it was devastated by the loss of two children in such a short time and it was presenting fatigue to prove it.

It was clear that this young woman would not get well while her mind and spirit were split apart, so I called on St. Johnswort to close the gap. The instant she received the St. Johnswort spirit, she sat bolt upright on the treatment table, her dull eyes suddenly gleaming. "Wow! I feel terrific!" she said. That was all it took to cure her fatigue.

In the beginning I used to have homeopathic preparations made of each plant I used as medicine, and these preparations served as a carrier to deliver the healing spirits to my patients. Later on I began to use the services of *erodium cicutarium,* otherwise known as filaree or storksbill.

Filaree is a pretty little plant commonly found in disturbed soil in temperate areas around the world. It has lacy fern-like leaves and magenta star-shaped flowers. The spirit of this plant offered itself to me as a kind of spiritual messenger service. I couldn't imagine why I would need a messenger until later, when the Food and Drug Administration cut off the supply of my homeopathic remedies. I returned to the filaree spirit and asked if it could summon the spirits of other plants I might need to help heal my patients. The spirit said it would be delighted to do this. It was hard for me to believe this would work, but I either had to take him at his word or abandon plant spirit medicine altogether. I took him at his word and found he delivers a purer, more specific medicine than the laboratory does.

Since that time I have experimented with various methods of preparing filaree to use in treatment: homeopathic potentization, radionics, flower essences and others. On some occasions I have asked my messenger to bring plant spirits through my hands into my patient's body. All these methods work well. Currently I most often give drops of filaree flower essence, asking my messenger to summon a specific plant spirit. I am certain that plain water would work just as well, because, after all, the magic is not in the matter. It's in the spirit.

Part III

Medicine Dreams
of the Shamans

Don Enrique Salmon

In the process of writing this book I confirmed something I had suspected since beginning my work with plants: I did not invent plant spirit medicine. All around the world there are shamans who heal with the spirits of plants. This is one of the great medical traditions of the planet.

Why have we never heard of plant spirit medicine before? Generations of ethnobotanists have catalogued the practices of plant healers in every corner of the earth, and yet there is no literature on their spiritual healing practices unless they happen to use "psychedelic" plants. Is the spirit bound to only a few psychoactive molecules? Will social scientists ever be able to admit that every plant is a miracle and a mystery? In looking for ways to avoid ecological cataclysm, will modern humanity take the time to learn from our plant brothers and sisters how to live successfully on the earth? If we do so soon, we may find that there are still a few plant shamans left who can introduce us to vegetable wisdom.

In this section of the book, we will meet five such people. Each has his or her own way of relating to the spirit power of plants, yet each story elaborates on the same themes: dreams, pilgrimage and vision quest as the true sources of knowledge; the willingness of plant spirits to teach and heal humankind; the journey to the Underworld; the importance of individualized and "nonroutine" treatment of patients; the power and aliveness of the elements; and the importance of gratitude and humility.

Our first plant shaman is Enrique Salmon, a young man of a Mexican tribe known as the Raramuri, or the Tarahumara. Don Enrique grew up in Southern California and was trained in the traditions of his people by his parents and grandparents. Fluent in English, Spanish and Raramuri, he is uniquely well equipped to interpret ancient wisdom to modern people.

The interview that follows took place near his home in the American Southwest.

Eliot:	Tell me how you learned some of the things you know about plant spirits.
Enrique:	Well, growing up it was my grandparents being around and my Mom always teaching me things about plants. As a little kid, the way I was brought up, we used plants instead of going to a doctor for healing. I was told by my grandparents when I was about twelve that they were going to teach me about plants. I did not really care about it at the time. I was busy with other things, just being a kid. But they started teaching me.
Eliot:	So your training as a shaman started with plants?
Enrique:	Yes. What plants are good for—what illnesses and that sort of thing. They waited for a while, until I got a little more mature before they started to be concerned with how to get in touch with the spirits within the plants. They taught me certain songs and certain ways to pick the plants and to pray to the plants and the earth, to bring out more of the medicine in a plant.
Eliot:	And that's what the songs were for?
Enrique:	The songs are to the plants and to the Earth also, to get the medicine out of the plant to help the patient more. Asking the plant for its help. Asking for it to do what it naturally does, for what it was put here for. As I got older I kept learning different things and eventually my grandfather started to teach me more about spiritual healing—how to get in touch with the spirits that are around us all the time and those spirits that get inside of someone who is possessed by a spirit or from a witch or a sorcerer. I learned about that. I learned about protecting those people and then healing those people with the use of the spirits. Because the spirits are out there just waiting to help us. We've got to use the right words or the songs to get them to help out a little. So I learned that for a while, until I was eighteen. Then I moved away from home. By that time I was fairly accomplished, but I still had a lot to learn.
	I picked up some more when I was in New Mexico on the Navajo land. They talked more about divination. It

was a different technique to tell what is wrong with a person. Then this Oglala Sioux guy taught me a lot about the four directions and how to be in contact with those spirits. Then frequent trips down into Chihuahua and learning some more by watching and asking a lot of questions with healers down there. So that is pretty much the extent of my education that got me here so far.

I am still learning. I still pick up things. I am still asking a lot of questions. I guess it's a practice just like other practices. If you don't practice for a while, you kind of miss some of your power. I haven't had a chance to do much around here. In Colorado I had a lot of people who were always asking me to help them out. I was pretty popular there as a healer. I just haven't had a chance around here. I feel like someone who is getting a little weak, you know?

Eliot: I'm sure it will come back when you need it.

Enrique: Oh yeah! Well, my mind has been on other things, too, like school and all that. It's like lifting weights. You keep on lifting weights or you will lose your strength a little bit. That's how I look at it.

Eliot: Is there anything you would like to say about specific individual plants? How you used them to help other people? What you have learned from them?

Enrique: My plant spirit helper is what we call *chuchupate* or the Mexicans call it *osha*. It is a very powerful plant, but also a very forgiving plant. What I mean is, some plants are very strong as medicine, but they have all these side effects. Osha is not like that at all. It is very strong, but it doesn't do anything to you on the side. I use it for infections, cuts, arthritis, headaches, sore throats, colds, stomach aches. It cures almost anything. You make a strong tea or just take the root and chew it. It tastes awful. I always carry a piece with me. It repels rattlesnakes and witches. You have to watch out for those witches. You never know when they are going to be around the next corner. Osha talks to me sometimes.

Eliot: Does it?

Enrique: Yes. The root. The whole plant will talk, but I get more messages from the root. In order to talk to the root you have to dig it up out of the ground, but it stays alive. Even when it dries out, it's still alive. You can take that dried up root after a year, put it in a glass of water and it will come back to life. You replant it and it will grow. A very tough, very determined plant.

Eliot: What are the things it says to you?

Enrique: It helps me figure out what is wrong with people. If I have a problem with a patient and I'm not quite sure what to do, I can go to osha. It will tell me. It will help me figure out what plants it can work with. Also, osha will let me know when I am getting in too deep in a problem.

Eliot: Someone else's problem or your own?

Enrique: Someone else's problems do become my own, especially when I am working with spells, when people have become possessed by something. Osha will tell me, "Hey, take it easy here!" or it will help me figure out how to go about a ceremony. There was one instance where a woman had a bad back. She went to doctors and they could not do anything, so she came to me. Osha told me to do something I have never done before or since: to draw this particular design on the ground and have her sit on it. I can't even remember what this drawing was any more. I know it had a big circle with little half circles around it. So that's one way osha will help out. Sometimes it will say, "You can't help this person. You are not strong enough yet." So it is my plant spirit helper.

Eliot: How do you go about putting yourself into the state of mind to receive those communications from plants?

Enrique: I try and find a quiet place to relax for a few hours. I can do it at home, but it's better outside. I'm not really thinking much about other things. I will drink some of the tea from the plant and get the plant itself. This is what is weird: I work with plants that have been picked. The spirits inside stay alive. I drink some of the tea, then I wait for something to happen. I'll do it right before I go to sleep, and wait for a dream. Or I will do it in the middle of the day and sit there and hum a little medicine song. I close my eyes and the spirit will come to me. It really doesn't look like a person to me. Usually it's animals. The animal will come and I hear the voice in Raramuri say, "Hi, how are you doing? This is who I am. Do you have any questions?" I will ask the question and they will answer. Sometimes they say, "Oh, I can't tell you that right now," or "You are not ready for that right now," or "Maybe when you are fifty years old. Right now you are too young," or something like that. They are generally good messages that help me to figure out how to use a plant. Sometimes they don't tell me much of anything. But it's always a very positive experience.

Eliot: Is that a method you developed yourself or did your grandfather show you how to do it?

Enrique: My grandmother showed me her way of doing it, which is different. She would talk to the live plants, touch them, and just sit there. I developed this other way because I was in the service, then I was in college. I didn't always have the time to go out into the countryside to meet the plants. That's where I found the spirits are still in the plants after you picked them and they dried up. Not for very long though. Maybe after eight months they are not there any more. I incorporated the chanting. That is something I learned from my grandfather; he always used to sing. So I incorporated what I learned from both my grandparents. It's just something that works for me—very powerful.

Eliot: When you are using the healing power of plants spirits, do you always have your patient eat or drink some part of the plant?

Enrique: Sometimes the spirits will tell me to combine certain plants to use as a smoking ritual.

Eliot: For you to smoke?

Enrique: Yes, for me to smoke and blow onto the patient. The spirit of the plant comes out in a visible form and goes into the patient to make them stronger.

Eliot: Have you done healing at a distance with plant spirits?

Enrique: Using corn, I have done healing at a distance. There was a friend of mine, can't remember what tribe he was from, who was going to court one day and he asked me the night before if I would do something to make the situation at court a positive one for everyone. He told me the time they were going to meet at this court place and at the same time I went outside using corn meal and a couple of songs. Corn is a very positive plant, healing all sorts of ways, so I used the corn to make things good there. It worked. Everybody came out winning. He said when it was all over, they came out still friends. To this day things still work out.

Eliot: What about songs? Have the plants taught you any songs?

Enrique: Yes. The plants have taught me a few songs. I forgot a couple of them. They were songs I used for a particular instance. There is one general song that I was taught that I use all the time in working with plants.

Eliot: It was taught by?

Enrique: By my grandfather. It is a very simple song. Tarahumara songs are redundant. The people in the ceremony get restless because I keep on repeating it. When I sing the song right now it's not going to do anything; it has to be in a different situation. ["Hey Hey Hey Hey."] That's it. It's just the spirit of the song that I learned from my grandfather. It's a general cure-all song. There are some more specific songs for other occasions. Like when I'm healing a place or a whole family—that song is like, "Hey Ya Ho Ya Hey Ya Ho." It keeps on repeating like that.

I've got a lot of bugs on my legs. It must be the cream I put on.

Eliot: I've got a few of them, too.

Enrique: They are always after me. I must have good medicine or something. I'm trying to remember a plant song. Listen to this—it is not a typical Tarahumara song at all: "Hey Hey Hey Hey." That one was in conjunction with sagebrush. The sage was telling me to sing this song. I was using it for a spiritual cleansing on a friend of mine. He had a hard time. For a while there he had these witches after him. I used that song a lot. I haven't used it since he left. I guess it was just a song for him.

You have to be careful with plants. Some of those herb books you buy in the beginning, they say, "Here is some information, but you should always consult a doctor or a herbologist—someone who knows what they are doing." There is a big health food store in Colorado with a big herb section in jars and packets. This woman who was a customer was talking to the resident herbologist. She was saying she had all these symptoms. She was always tired, always felt weak, could never sleep, things like that. So this herbologist named off seven different plants—plants that I would never dream of using next to each other. The customer was going to spend about a hundred dollars on these herbs. After the herbologist left, I went up to her and said, "Save your money." She was like, "Who are you?" because I don't look like a healer, I guess. What exactly does a healer look like? I think Americans have this idea about shamans, especially what they look like. I don't know about you, but I guess you look like a lawyer or a CPA.

Eliot: Somebody accused me of looking like a computer technologist.

Enrique: Maybe it's the glasses. So, anyway, she is looking at me and saying, "Who are you?" I said, "Don't waste your money on all these plants. Just go home and start eating right and exercising and from that you will start sleeping better and when you sleep better, you won't be so tired. Go ahead and drink a lot of cota and spearmint. That's all you need." I'm not sure what she did.

To me, that herbologist is an example of someone who is taking advantage of what they think they know. Perhaps she took a few classes or read a bunch of books. It takes more than that. I have been doing it since I was twelve and still I don't profess to know everything. There is no way to know everything. You are always learning until you die. She might not have caused that woman too much harm except for her pocketbook, but some people actually hurt people with what they are doing.

Eliot: Is there anything else you want to talk about?

Enrique: For a long time, I would only work with Native Americans and Hispanics because I thought they understood where I was coming from, that would make it work. If someone comes in off the street who has always gone to whiteman doctors and they want me to heal them using spirit medicine, it probably is not going to work, or that's what I thought for a long time. But then I had a vision. I was on a medicine quest three years ago, on the side of this mountain range by myself, seeking some more medicine, some more ideas—singing songs and smoking things—nothing hallucinogenic, just smoking certain plants and waiting for something to happen. A bear was hanging around a lot, but he was just there to protect me from what might harm me because I was there by myself. I was getting a lot of messages from the deer. Finally it came to me in a dream from the deer that I was not going to get any new medicine from this quest. "What I'm going to give you is a path to follow. Not a new path, but something to add on to the path you are on already." It was to pass on some approaches to the spirit world for white people. Native Americans have their way of finding out things. If a big storm comes along, Native Americans' roots are deep into the earth. We are still going to be here. But for a lot of Anglos, there aren't many roots. The next storm comes along and they would all be blown off the universe. I was told to help out these people any way I can: how to approach the spirit world, how a Native American develops roots into the earth. The only way I can think about how to do it is what we are doing right now. Tell people how to go about learning things. How I get messages from the plants, from the spirits. Maybe someone can read your book and learn a few more things, a few more ideas. Because the traditions are missing.

My way isn't going to work for everybody. The Tarahumara ways aren't going to work for white people or Apaches or whatever because there is this mind set that comes with traditions. I think that the best way for Anglos is not to adopt our traditional ways, but to learn from us how traditions work. Then put these together and say, "Okay, how does this work? How can this work for us?"

Eliot: I guess that's basically what I'm doing.

Enrique: Yeah! Yeah! That's why I like what you are up to.

Eliot: A typical white person, if he wants to learn something about plants, will go to a university and read a lot of books and listen to lectures of other people who have read books.

Enrique: That is a different way of knowing.

Eliot: That's right! I would like you to talk a little bit about your way of knowing.

Enrique: I am sort of an enigma myself.

Eliot: I mean the knowing of your people.

Enrique: Okay. To a Tarahumara, knowing something has nothing to do with being able to use the scientific name of the plant. Americans like to put everything in their own little boxes. For the Tarahumara or Raramuri everything interconnects; you can't really put something into its own little box. That would be to kill it, to cut it off. It has these big root systems throughout the universe. To take one part of this root system and put it in a box to classify it is to kill it. Everything is interconnected.

Eliot: How does a Tarahumara go about learning about plants?

Enrique: We Tarahumaras have our basic education as we are growing up. It has nothing to do with reading books. We learn how to use particular plants for healing, for food, for drinks. We're taught by example. Taught about how to farm particular plants. Now, if a Tarahumara wants to learn a little bit more than the average person, he has to get in contact with the spirits and wait for a dream. That dream takes him into the real world. We don't live in the real world here. This is a flesh and blood world, not the real world. The real world is where the spirit of osha comes and talks to me. The real world isn't in the technology or all those books. It's in our visions and dreams. Whenever we dream or have a vision, a door is opening for us. If we learn something from that, that's when we actually know something. That is "knowing." That's how it works. If I want to know more than the normal Tarahumara knows, I have to experience that through visions and dreams. Not every Tarahumara does that. We are born with different paths. Some of us were made to be good farmers. Some of us are put here to be healers. Some are put here to be good basket-makers.

Some Tarahumaras have become Christians or Catholics. Those that become Catholics, that is no big deal. Catholicism is really cool because it does sort of ritualize. That ritual takes you to this other realm and so that's good. Jehovah's Witnesses and Protestants take the Tarahumara away from the real knowing, because knowing to the Christians is this book—the Bible. But knowing is not in the written words, not in the book. That is what scientists do. Traditional Tarahumaras still respect this other way of knowing things. Some Tarahumaras will travel days to go to a person he respects to have that person help them out to learn things.

Eliot: Are these "knowers" the most respected people among the Tarahumara?

Enrique: Yes! They are the older people who have been around for a while who have taken the time to learn these things and to pass this information on and keep traditions around. I was thinking about my mom, for example. She didn't finish school, but she is one of the wisest people I know. If someone from the University were to categorize her, she would be at the bottom of the list. But that is in White Man's society. If I were to take her to Hopi, for example, where they still respect the old ways, she would be considered a very intelligent person, very wise, because she knows a lot in that tradition. They would look at her and say, "Gosh, she can cook traditional foods. Take them right out of the earth. She doesn't need to go to Safeway. She can make these baskets. She knows about all these medicines." What more could you ask for? That's great! That is a lifetime of learning!

Most Americans don't understand that other sense of knowledge. Knowledge to Americans is being able to recite Shakespeare from memory, to split up an atom, or something like that. But what does that do for you except being able to write papers to impress these other people who don't know what they're talking about either? I'm getting my Ph.D., but those three little letters are not going to make me a stronger healer. They are not going to help me learn more about herbs or be able to pick corn off the stalk and make it into tortillas. All it's going to do is when I write articles or a book, people are going to be willing to read it. It is kind of sad.

Eliot: I wanted to ask you about something entirely different. Do you have anything to say about using local plants versus using plants that grow somewhere else?

Enrique: When I'm healing someone, I prefer to use plants from the area where the person lives. A person living in this area is in contact with these plants around them. These plants are affecting them and they don't realize it. These plants are tough. They send out these messages. A lot of the people that have been here for a long time, they seem like the plants out here. They are tough people. They realize it's a tough environment, but they endure it because they love it. It becomes a part of them. So that's why I like to use plants from a person's environment as much as I can. Even have the person pick the plants that I'm going to use in the ceremony. I think it helps them feel the medicine spirit of the plant to know where the medicine is coming from. A lot of white man medicines, you don't know where it comes from. It comes from some lab. Sometimes they do come from the plants, but they pretty much killed the spirit of the plant by the time they turn it into a pill or some liquid in a jar. The chemicals are there, I guess, but they are not live chemicals. In that sense, I try to use most plants from their environment.

Don Lucio Campos

It was the Indian herbalist, Doña Modesta, who told me where Don Lucio Campos lives. I had taken my friend John to Doña Modesta's house for treatment. He lay on a mat in the sun while she prayed over him and rubbed fresh herbs into his skin. When the healing was over, my friend rested quietly while Doña Modesta and I chatted.

"People from your country come here wanting me to teach them about herbs," she said, "but they are always looking for herbs to treat certain diseases. They say, 'And this disease, Doña Modesta, what plant is there for this disease?' I tell them, 'There are no herbs for specific illnesses.' Then they say, 'There has to be a plant for this problem.' So I tell them, 'Well, if there has to be a plant for this problem, then go out and find it yourself!'"

Modesta laughed, and continued, "I use the same plants for everything: the same ones my mother used. When she was alive, she was the best healer in the village; now I am the best."

"Doña Modesta," I asked her, "how much of the healing is performed by the spirit of the plants?"

"A lot. The juice of the plants is their blood. The blood captures the healing power of the sun. When I pick them, our brothers the plants sacrifice themselves to share that power with us."

"Doña, I am learning a little bit about plant medicine myself, but my mother did not teach me, as yours did. I learn by chatting with plants."

"You do?"

"Yes. Don't you talk with plants?"

"Of course!" she confided with a wink. "But I don't tell my students that!"

"Why not?"

"Some of them wouldn't believe me."

"Listen, Doña, have you ever heard of a healer called Don Lucio?"

"Yes. I know him. He lives near Tlalnepantla. They call him 'the shaman.'"

"I have heard that he heals with plant spirits, that he does not use leaves or flowers. They say he invokes the plant spirits just by calling their names."

"I don't believe in that kind of thing. No, the blood of the plants is what heals. You've got to get it onto the body—the brain, the heart, the spine, the liver, the kidneys. You have to get the juice of the plants close to the important organs!"

After Doña Modesta told me where to find him, I went to meet Don Lucio myself. Arriving at his house, I found out that he was entertaining a Guatemalan herbalist and his two apprentices. They were all on their way to take the sheep to graze. I caught up with them in the road beside the corral. The old shaman had saddled his horse and was standing there holding the reins.

The Guatemalan herbalist was standing on tiptoes with a freshly-picked plant in one hand. His other hand was cupped to his mouth. "And, this?" he shouted into Don Lucio's ear. "What do they call this plant in your language, in Nahuatl?"

Don Lucio pronounced the name.

The Guatemalan shouted back, "In Quiché, my language, we call this...." He made a softly guttural sound. "And here in Mexico, what medicinal use do you make of this plant?"

"I didn't know that this was medicinal!"

"Yes, compadre, this is medicinal!"

"Ah, imagine that! I had no idea! And what do you use it for?"

"This plant is good for old people when they are deaf like yourself," shouted the herbalist. "You let it dry in the sun for two or three hours and then you stuff it in your ears."

"Oh, so this is medicinal!" said Don Lucio good-naturedly.

We set out into the countryside with Don Lucio on horseback leading his sheep on a winding trail and the Guatemalans and myself walking down the roadway. Whenever the herbalist saw a plant he recognized he would stop, pick a stalk, and briefly explain to his students how to use it. Our progress was very slow; the teacher seemed to know everything that grew along the way. I was not privy to these lessons, as the three men spoke to each other in their own language.

Whenever Don Lucio's path crossed our own, the teacher would accost him in Spanish:

"Compadre, what do you call this plant in Nahuatl?"

The apprentices would scribble down Lucio's reply.

"Compadre, in Quiché we call this…[another soft guttural sound]. And do you use this for food or medicine?" the Mayan would ask.

"No, I don't know any use for this."

"This is medicine, compadre! This is wonderful for…" (and he would name an affliction).

"Oh, so this is a medicine, then! Imagine that! I had no idea!" The old man seemed to enjoy admitting his ignorance as much as the younger one relished displaying his knowledge. Both of them seemed quite happy with themselves by the time we returned to Don Lucio's home.

Don Lucio invited me into his parlor. The Guatemalans excused themselves, and I never saw them again.

The parlor was filled with the fragrance of freshly cut flowers. An entire wall was taken up by an elaborate altar filled with crucifixes, images of saints, and the like. The rest of the room was bare, save for five or six straight-backed chairs. The shaman motioned me to sit in one chair, and took another next to mine.

He turned to me with a smile and clapped his hand on my knee. "Well, my boy, what can we do for you?"

"I do healing with plants," I said, "but I use the spirit of the plants, not the flesh." I put my hand on his forearm. "I understand that you do something similar."

"What?" he said.

I cupped my hand to my mouth, leaned over close to his ear, and shouted, "I use plant spirits to heal people. You do too?"

"Yes! The spirits of the plants! That's it! Plants have movement! They have spirit! They even have soul! If not, they wouldn't be alive; the Lord wouldn't have put them here!"

"When you heal people, you don't make them eat or drink their medicine?"

"No! I do my work purely with intention!" He tapped his forehead with his index finger.

"There are very few of us who work that way," I said.

"Yes! Not like these people from Guatemala who go around looking for substances! This is the way I work…." Here Don Lucio launched into a complicated story, using his free hand to touch mine at moments of particular interest. The gist of the story was how he used magical means to free a man he had never met from unjust imprisonment in a faraway city. After his release, the man traveled to Don Lucio's village to offer thanks. The two men met by accident in the street. Lucio had no idea who the visitor was, but the visitor recognized Lucio immediately.

From his prison cell window he had seen the shaman coming to his rescue. "That's the way it is," the old man concluded. "That's the way it works."

"How did you learn what you know?" I asked him.

"No one taught me. When I was quite young I was struck by lightning. I had walked out in the country by myself. I saw the lightning coming down at me. It was like a ball, all different colors, very beautiful! Then it hit me and I lost consciousness. I was on the ground for over two hours; it was no laughing matter! Then I got up and went home, but I was very sick. I would go into coma, then come to for a few minutes, and then go back again. In all, I was in bed for three years. When my body was lying there, my soul was traveling and learning!

"The first year I spent with the Weather People in the heavens. I traveled all over the earth with the Weather People, to every country, bringing rain. The second year I spent with the Seeds. I met the spirit of all the plants that are cultivated by humankind. The third year I spent with the Flocks and the Herding People. I met all the different kinds of herding animals. I've been everywhere! I've seen it all! The Italians! The Eskimos! The Russians! The Africans! And you know, we are all brothers! You are my brother because the blood that flows in my veins also flows in yours! Isn't that so?"

"Yes, Don Lucio, that's the way it is...." We exchanged a glance. "You know, Don Lucio, once when I was at the pyramid of El Tepozteco, I met the Rain God." Intimidated by the Catholic images on his altar, I did not dare mention the god's pagan name.

"Tlaloc!" he said.

"Yes, Tlaloc! He taught me many things. I saw him with streams of water flowing from the palms of his hands."

"Of course! He's the one who hands out the water to this world. That's why I have him here with me. When it is dry and I ask for rain so that my people don't have to suffer, I have to have someone to back me up. So I keep Tlaloc with me."

"Wait a minute! You mean you have Tlaloc on your altar?"

"Naturally! Come, I'll show you." He took his hand off my knee and lead me to the shrine.

Crowded amongst other religious images on the table, there stood a carved wooden mask of Jesus. He removed the mask to reveal a grotesque stone idol of the Nahuatl Rain God Tlaloc.

We went back to our chairs and resumed our embrace. "How old do you think I am?" he asked.

Judging him to be about seventy-five, I said, "Oh, I don't know, maybe sixty-five."

"You didn't miss by much, my friend. I turned seventy-eight last September seventh. And yet, I still like the ladies! Now why do you suppose that is?" he grinned.

"Just natural, I suppose."

"Just natural, eh? Are you married, my boy?"

"Yes. I have children."

"Ah, I tell you my friend, this world is like no other. This is the only place you can make love and make lots of babies. The Lord wanted His people to be many, not just a puny few scattered here and there! That's why he made the world this way.

"But this world can be difficult, too. People do bad things to each other. Envy. It makes for a lot of illness, you know. It's terrible the things that people do to each other. Then I have to remove the illness people cause each other with their envy.

"This is not the only world, though. There is another world besides this one! The other world is beautiful, my brother! The food there is great! Not just tiny little bits like in this world; there you can eat huge amounts! You can make love all the time, and no babies! There is no fatigue! Your body is light like a feather! That world is beautiful. And that is where healing comes from. That's the way it is, brother, and that's how my work is: beautiful!"

"Thank you, Don Lucio," I say. "It has been a real pleasure meeting you. I will come back and see you again soon. And if you ever find yourself in my town, my house is yours."

"Thank you. I will be waiting for your next visit. And when you return, bring me one of those American girls. A good one!"

When I returned, I brought no American girls, but Don Lucio made no mention of that. He was busy preparing for a ceremony. A neo-Aztec group occupied his parlor: clouds of incense poured from the door and windows. Ceremonialists dressed in pre-Columbian costumes played lutes and sang in praise of the Star of Bethlehem and the Way of the Cross.

I entered the parlor. I was addressed by a bearded athletic-looking man in a silver lamé loincloth and a three-foot-high plumed headdress. He asked me to remove my hat, which I did. I had heard this ceremony was to honor Tlaloc, so I had brought an offering of chocolate. I handed it to a priestess, who passed it through incense smoke, offered it to the four directions, and placed it at the altar among the other offerings, which were all of flowers.

I walked outside, to find Don Lucio looking a trifle impatient.

"Where will your ceremony be held?" I asked.

"As soon as these people are done," he answered, "I will lead everyone to the church."

Obviously my intelligence had been wrong. This event could not be in honor of Tlaloc. No pagan god would be honored in a Catholic church. I wondered what kind of ceremony Don Lucio would give.

After a long wait, the old man picked up two baskets of flowers and set out towards the village church. I followed behind, lugging a heavy five-foot candle he had asked me to carry.

The church was decorated with hundreds of candles, thousands of flowers and lots of colored paper. It was the festival of La Candelaria: Jesus, Light of the World. Scarcely had Lucio placed his offerings before the altar when the Aztec troupe marched in with censers smoking. They placed themselves in formation before the altar and began to chant loudly. Village people started arriving. A contingent of young girls in luxurious white first communion dresses took their place next to the semi-naked Aztecs. The village priest walked up to the altar and put on his vestment. Before long a throng of faithful filled the church and spilled out onto the steps of the entrance. Mass was celebrated. The Aztecs began a parting song. They backed out of the church with military precision, still singing and playing their instruments. By the time they got to the courtyard, the village brass band was already blaring a spicy tune, and skyrockets were exploding in booming clusters. Vendors were hawking candy and soft drinks. The girls in the white dresses flocked out, giggling. A couple of violinists sawed away at a dance tune, unheard in the din. It was the typical Mexican chaos, and nothing at all to do with Tlaloc—or so I thought. I left without saying good-bye to Don Lucio.

I drove home under the usual clear blue skies, for it was the second of February—the height of the dry season. That night I was awakened by claps of thunder announcing a downpour. When I got up the next morning, the town was soaked and the sky was faultlessly blue, promising many more weeks of sunny weather. I thought of Don Lucio's altar, where the Rain God stands hidden behind a mask of Jesus Christ.

Sharon Puhky-Evans

Sharon Puhky-Evans is a housewife and mother of two who lives near Victoria, British Columbia. A few years ago, she enrolled in a local acupuncture college, and while a student there, she also trained with me in plant spirit medicine. As part of that training, she went on a spiritual pilgrimage, or vision quest. One year after the experience, Sharon wrote the following account:

I had never done anything like this before. I had read about it and had a lot of curiosity. I had spiritual experiences throughout my life, but always unexpectedly. This time, we were setting a date.

The Carmanah Valley was decided on. This is a beautiful virgin rain forest. The idea was to have a sweat lodge and spend the night. As the weekend grew closer, I had a lot of apprehension about the "spending the night" part. I had not spent the night by myself in a forest before.

I started with a three day fast. We were to fast for one day, so my way of thinking was "more is better." On the third day, we set off to the Valley. We arrived to find a lovely sweat lodge built by members of the group who had come earlier.

We heated the rocks and entered the lodge. This was a very moving experience for me. The heat, herbs and chanting all seemed to be the right blend. After the sweat we were to find ourselves a spot to camp—not together, but out of earshot from each other.

When I found my spot by the river, I set up my little pup tent. I had become friendly with the trees and plants first by offering tobacco. I crawled into my sleeping bag and lay there. About a half an hour later, I nearly flipped when I heard footsteps.

It was my husband coming to check on me.

I lay there until it became quite dark. I was scared. I couldn't hear anyone. Then I had a very calm feeling come over me like a wash of warm water. I realized the forest wouldn't hurt me. It was at this point that things really started to happen.

I don't remember waking up. I found myself hiding behind a tree by my tent, crouched down. My heart was pounding. I was watching a hooded figure in gray walk slowly up the path. It was dark, but I could see very well. The figure turned and looked at me. It was an old man with a kind face. I wasn't afraid then. He started to speak to me. Most of the dialogue I want to keep private, but at one point he counseled me on many things. He was describing a certain aspect of the human condition. He was emphasizing the eyes, telling me that the eyes of a person are the key to understanding them, as well as a clue to how much protection I need for myself.

He stopped and looked away so I could not see his face. When he turned again, it wasn't the same kind old man. What I saw scared me so badly I couldn't breathe. My heart was pounding. The face had become cold and hard...the eyes were insane. They looked to be made of steel, like ball bearings. I saw then how one's soul could be lost. Not a word was spoken. Just the look. I saw that this was my test. Had I been listening? Could I protect myself?

My next memory was of being awakened. It seemed that someone had the corner of my tent and was yanking it up and down. It was still dark. I turned around in my bag and could see through the tent wall. A very large white rabbit was sitting there. "Wake up!" I heard. The rabbit took two jumps and transformed itself into a sleek, wild cat. The cat turned and looked at me. "Not everything is what it seems," it said. It then ran off. The next thing I knew, it was morning.

Even as I write this now, I can tell you, this is a clear memory. But I'm sure you can understand my hesitation when Eliot asked me to share this story. If it hadn't happened to me, I don't know if I would believe it. Needless to say, it was quite a night!

About a year after she wrote this account, I interviewed Sharon to find out what fruit her vision had borne:

Eliot: Is there any part of the story of your vision quest that you left out last time that you feel OK about sharing now?

Sharon: Sure. The part that I left out was the instructions about how to protect my heart and how important that is. In working with people, through the eyes I can see what condition the soul is in. Before I even look, it's important to protect my heart. I do visualization to do that. I was told that I would meet all kinds of people. Without protection, I would be laying myself open to all kinds of problems. That was two years ago; that's the part I left out. I felt vulnerable after the vision quest. I didn't want it known that I needed to have my heart protected. So I left that out.

Eliot: Can you tell us something about how your work has developed as a result of your vision?

Sharon: Everything started to happen afterwards; none of this was happening before the vision quest. In plant spirit medicine, I didn't make a good connection with my messenger plant. The one that I made the real connection with was artemisia (mugwort). So when I went to treat a patient for the first time, I went to artemisia for help, and that's when the doors flung open.

Eliot: Will you describe that?

Sharon: OK. An elderly fellow came to me who had had open heart surgery ten years ago. I decided to do a treatment with plant spirit medicine because he was afraid of [acupuncture] needles. As I called for my protection, I realized that I didn't want him to see me. I stood behind him and put my hands on his head and asked him to close his eyes. When I called on my artemisia spirit, he was right there. I just watch what he does. It's like watching television.

Before I start, I say a prayer. I ask that the patient be helped with their heartfelt need, because you know people come and say, "This is the problem," but when you work down through the layers, you see that it's not the problem at all. So before I start, I say a prayer and I tell artemisia, "I have faith in whatever you are going to do."

Eliot:

So that is what you did this first time—and what happened?

Sharon:

It was incredible. I saw an exorcism take place. When I was interviewing this fellow, I was listening to his story and at the same time I was asking, "What does he really need?" The answer I got was, "He needs a sweet heart." He'd had grievous injury. He had a broken heart from a previous marriage.

Artemisia appears to me in a certain form—as a warrior. He has certain dress and rattles that he uses and a stick with feathers on it. There is a sacred fire that is very important because it does so many different things...the smoke from the artemisia fire. In this case, the smoke entered [the acupuncture points used to perform exorcism]. Then I saw a split in this person along the scar from his open heart surgery. The split opened and a large piece of cellophane came out. It had different images on it: darkness, figures, shadows. As it came up into the light, it was dissipating. Then the artemisia warrior came and did a rattling around the patient. I had never seen anything like that in my life.

So, after the treatment, I say my thank you's, and the artemisia warrior will tell me when it's over. Then I open my eyes and go wash my hands and come back.

This man sent me a card a month ago. I wish I had brought it. It's taped on my fridge.

Previous to that, the very first time I did this was a few months before with a client of mine. She had a strong treatment reaction to this. It brought up a lot of emotion and old memories. This kind of healing crisis is not uncommon when using the needles. She took herself to the hospital later that night. I was totally unprepared for what was going on. I learned a lot from her. So this time I prepared him. I told him, "Don't be surprised if you're tired or have disturbed sleep. Any thoughts that come up, just pay attention. It's all part of the treatment." Now I prepare people.

The card was just wonderful. He has come to see me since then and he invariably brings it up, "What was that that you gave me?" Anyway, when he came back after that first session, he said, "I feel like I have my heart. I feel like I have a sweet heart! I still have fatigue, but I don't worry about it. My heart feels full now!"

I see him every six weeks now. He was coming down for an operation on his chest because he had had X-rays, and there was a shadow on the X-ray. He was quite concerned. They had scheduled him for this exploratory surgery. He came the night before and asked me, "Could you do that again for me?" I said, "Sure."

Eliot: What had you been doing with him in between times?

Sharon: Acupuncture. So, anyway, I did this artemisia thing with him again. It was very nice. Totally different from the first time. It had to do with protecting him, cocooning him, cleaning him out. He went off to the hospital the next morning. He said that he went in for his X-ray, and he's all prepped for them to open him up, and there's nothing. The shadow is *gone* from his heart. His doctor says, "I don't know what happened. It was there in November. But we're not going to do this to you. You are elderly, and it's stressful, and there's no point." And he feels great! He's reduced his heart medication. So he sends me this card saying how much he appreciated my help. It's restored his faith in something. It was very nice.

Eliot: Tell us some more stories.

Sharon: Goodness, let's see…. The woman who was so frightened by her memories—she came back next time and she was really angry. She said "What was that?" She thought it was LSD. I said, "Of course not. I would never do something like that."

Eliot: What did she experience?

Sharon: She had all kinds of tumultuous emotions. She felt she was losing control.

Eliot: And what had you seen in her treatment?

Sharon: Just a lot of turmoil. I was just watching. This was not fun.

So, as we worked together with acupuncture, she realized that I was a good person and I was helping her. We developed communication. After four or five months, I said, "How would you feel if we gave this another try?" And she said "Yes." She didn't hesitate. She said, "Let's do it."

Next time I saw her, I did it. I did my asking for protection, and I asked for help, and gave my respect, and then, what I saw looked like a strand of pearls wrapped around her neck. As the pearls started to be pulled away from her neck, I realized that there was writing on each and every one of them. They weren't really pearls. They were tiny little bags tied up with string. On every one of them was written: "Tears and Hurt." The artemisia warrior just reached in and pulled them up to the sun and they disappeared. It was really moving for me to see that.

After I do this kind of thing, the room seems different to me. It becomes womb-like—soft and muted. There is a feeling between the person and me. This time it was really, really wonderful. She looked at me and said, "Thank you." She really meant it. I thought, "You're welcome!" I went to wash my hands and come back.

I went to touch her neck, and her whole body had turned red. She said she felt like she had been hit by a lightning bolt. I took her pulses, and her pulses were wonderful. I went and got Dr. Hong, who was my supervisor at the time. He came in and looked at her. Then, he looked at me. He picked up her hand and said, "She's done."

This woman got up and left. He called me into his office. I thought I was in trouble because he thought I had treated her with acupuncture without supervision. I said, "I didn't needle her." He said, "No, you sure didn't. Well, what did you do?" I said, "I just touched her neck." He said, "Before you did that, what did you do?" I said, "I gave her this little herbal tincture. It's completely benign." He said, "I want you to write this case up!"

Afterwards, the patient calls me up and tells me that her doctor sent her to have blood work done. Then the doctor calls me and says that her blood chemistry is normal. Its never been this good. "Whatever it was, you're doing real good work." That was kind of exciting! As this was the first client I had treated in this manner, feedback was very important.

At the time this happened with this client, I was finishing my third year at the school, which was a supervised clinic. I was very fortunate to have Dr. Hong as my supervisor. He is, in my opinion, the best teacher there. He was competent, kind and supportive. I started to use this work in my preliminary treatments with my clients. It very quickly became the most important part of the treatment plan, as it enable me to learn so much more about my client. What would normally take me hours to do with the needles, Artemisia would do in a few brief moments. With the information he would give me, I would draw up the treatment plan. He hasn't been wrong yet. This is very important, as I am very much a skeptic. What he tells me is the client's story, not mine. I do edit information now. Some of this work is very scary and can be very gross, but the outcome is always good. Artemisia can take care of anything. I mean, *anything.*

Something very important has happened from me in this work. As I've said before, I am a very skeptical person. I don't have guru. I don't go off to India looking for whatever. I have always felt connected to life. I have certainly had my share of difficulties, but when I really needed solace, I went to my garden. This is where I would pour out my troubles and fill my heart. This has always worked for me, even as a child. Who could imagine that those plants heard me? Amazing! So I feel really at home with this work. I have a lot of questions still, but it doesn't seem so strange to me anymore. My faith is strengthened as my experience grows. We live in a world that we don't know much about, yet we find all we need here. Remember I told you about the "Man in Grey" from the Carmanah? Well, he told me things then that I didn't really believe at the time. As time has progressed, however, the list he gave me has checked out. One of the things he said was that my whole life as I knew it was about to change because of deception and betrayal (he meant my marriage) and that this work was going to become very important to me. This work was going to be the well spring of my own healing. Guess what? He was right! This is where I come now for my healing (you, Linda and Don Lupe). I'm a very lucky person. I make mistakes, but seem to land on my feet with a lot of help.

The bottom line here is: Does my client feel better? Are the things that are troubling to this person diminishing, easing up, going away? That is what I think this is all about. One time I asked Artemisia why he appeared in this form. He said that I wasn't that keen on the "white rabbit" and laughed. There is a lot of humor here, as well as the heavy stuff. The other night I saw a TV program about a Pharma-researcher going to the Amazon to talk to shamans about plants. I think I understand now how these people know their medicines. It's like this: we are really getting our medicine from plants. In this work, we just cut out the middle man and go straight to the source. You know, I wasn't a practitioner at first. Look what happened. Thanks for your support.

Eliot: I love to hear about this…. I love to hear about people who have developed their own relationship to the plant spirits. I think that's the way it should be done.

Sharon: Really?

Eliot: There is no better source of information than your experience and your patients' experience. Besides, there isn't anything else. There is this whole world tradition of people who are doing what we are doing, but for some reason it has been totally ignored. There is nothing in print.

Sharon: I know. I have looked.
One part of me gets anxious. "Maybe I'm not doing this right. Maybe there is some ritual to follow." Even though it's working just fine.

Eliot: Your spirits are there to help you. If they want you to do something differently, ask them to let you know. But if they are happy with what you are doing, who is there to tell you differently?

Sharon: No one, I guess…. I do have a lot of faith, because I get feedback. I'm careful to double check. When you have an X-ray and the shadow is gone, when the sed rate

	drops, when your blood work changes—you can't fake those things. You can't manipulate them.
Eliot:	While we're talking, let me just get this out of the corner.... I want to give you this—a magic wand made out of artemisia stems.
Sharon:	Oh no, really? Are you serious?
Eliot:	Yeah.
Sharon:	The artemisia warrior uses something just like this, but it has feathers on the top.
Eliot:	Yeah. I put feathers on the top sometimes.
Sharon:	You're kidding me!
Eliot:	I'm serious. I didn't know exactly why I made this thing. Maybe its for you.... Here.
Sharon:	For Heaven's sake! He uses something like this, with feathers on top!
Eliot:	Is it that long?
Sharon:	Yes, just like this. He uses it for cleansing. Incredible! An artemisia wand.... (laughs) That's it! I'm amazed! I've never seen anything like that before in real life.
Eliot:	Well, as they say, use it in the best of health! Sharon, has this treatment of yours ever failed to work so far?
Sharon:	No. All I have to do is ask, and it's right there. You know, I'm going down a totally different route than what I thought I would be. I feel like I'm on a roller coaster. You never know what is around the corner. Ever since I had the vision, my life has changed. I never know what I'm going to see. I've done this treatment for friends, for my ex-husband, for people I don't know, and it doesn't matter. It always works. It's always something different. That is probably a good thing, because I get bored easily! I never imagined.... I'm still awed.
Eliot:	I'm really happy to hear all this!
Sharon:	Every once in a while I find myself thinking, "What would have happened if I hadn't gone on that vision quest?" I feel like I would still be in the Dark Ages. That was the highlight of my decade, next to the birth of my children.

I've never done psychic work for people, but I feel that psychic work is another story entirely. It's one thing to have someone tell you what they saw, but with this, I can actually do something about it! I can actually help! I feel like I've really been given a gift—a bigtime gift. I feel really grateful. I want to thank you again for taking me up there. I would never have done anything like this on my own. I would probably have been afraid something like this would happen!

I saw Sharon again several months after our interview, and I asked her for a treatment. I was hoping that her spirits could help me with low back pain that had bothered me for many years.

She had me lie down on a massage table, and without further preliminaries she turned her back to me and faced the wall. Within a few seconds, I began to feel delicious surges of energy coursing through my body, particularly in the spine and pelvis. Washes of color crossed my visual field. After ten minutes or so, the sensations subsided and Sharon turned around to face me. The treatment was over. More than two years have gone by since that session, and I have been free of back pain ever since.

Tobae Agbaga Ason

I have never been to Australia or Asia, so I cannot document the existence of plant spirit medicine on those continents, because as Sharon Puhky-Evans and I discovered, there is no literature on the subject. This does not necessarily mean that the medicine does not exist. It is very easy to miss what you are not looking for, and evidently no one has been looking for it. Perhaps a few writers and scholars may read this book and realize that there is such a thing as plant spirit medicine. Then I am sure they will find it everywhere they look, just as I have.

I am happy to say that I do have a report from West Africa: plant spirit medicine is thriving there. My friend Siri Gian Singh Khalsa spent several years in Togo researching a doctoral thesis on medical practices in that country. I visited him at his home in Sacramento, California and asked him to share what he learned:

Eliot: You went to West Africa, to Togo. How long ago?

Siri: I was there from 1980 to 1984. I was comparing the history of traditional medicine and western medicine in Togo. Primarily I was focusing on the twentieth century. I tried to take my story as far back as I could go with the traditional healers.

Eliot: What did you discover about the role of herbs and plant spirits in traditional African healing?

Siri: The herbs were used in every facet of healing. There was a spirit associated with each herb that created the healing. Sounds were used to invoke those spirits in different plants. They also went into altered states through trance and sometimes through chemical means to have access to the information that the herbs could give them.

Certain people had trained as long as twenty years in order to hear the spirits of the herbs talking to them.

Eliot: Is this something that has a long lineage?

Siri: Yes. A friend of mine, Dr. Meerick Posnansky, one of the premier archaeologists of Africa, has found that one of the best ways to find villages that were in existence six, seven, eight hundred years ago is to go anywhere in Africa and find where their herbs encircle something, then dig inside where those herbs are—that would be the village. Many of the most widely used herbs would be grown secretly or openly around the village so that they could have access to these really crucial plants. There are instances where we can prove that certain herbs were used thousands of years ago. According to the traditions in the communities I studied, their herbal use goes back thousands of years.

Eliot: It is not necessarily the leaf or the root or the body of the plant that is used in the healing, but the spirit or essence of the plant. Is that right?

Siri: Yes, that is right! Each part of the plant had different qualities of spirit and there was also an overall plant spirit. The healers paid attention to both. So bark from one plant would be used for one purpose and the flower for another purpose and the leaf for another purpose just as western botanists do.

Eliot: Do you have any stories to tell about healings that you saw specifically involving plant spirits?

Siri: Every time there was a healing there were plants involved. Each plant had to be communicated with a specific way. Sounds of drums or voice would always be used to quicken the spirit of the plant. Something had to be done over the herbs in order to activate them and to make that herb an ally to the patient.

Eliot: Were you able to follow up on any cases?

Siri: Yes. Since I was studying with Western doctors and going to one of the most conservative institutions in the United States, the medical history department at UCLA, I had to include Western opinions of what was happening. I had hundreds of interviews with Western doctors and thousands of interviews with traditional healers.

The medical doctors would tell me about the illness of people they were treating. Many people who had been diagnosed and treated by western doctors would let me accompany them to traditional healers. I would get to see what herbs were given and how they were administered. What I found was that people who had diabetes—and we don't cure diabetes in the west, we just control it—that the herbs would be used to cure diabetes. When they would go back to the doctor, there would be no sign whatsoever of diabetes. Cancers, heart problems, a tremendous range of problems were diagnosed by the western practitioners and then treated by the traditional practitioners. Sometimes I would have to pay the person to go back to the medical doctor. They felt that they were okay, so why would they waste their time? I would want to have the validation by the physician, who sometimes would be very surprised. The older doctors were Africans who had studied at the University of Paris Medical School or the University of Lyons Medical School in France. The younger M. D.'s were very scathing and critical of the "superstitious, primitive, useless ways of the traditional healers." The older medical doctors who were African were always in respect of those ways because they had learned the limits of what they could do. They had seen that the African healers could cure things they could only hope to control at best. Maybe kill the pain, but not to cure. There developed a real interaction between the two systems. Everybody that I interviewed in this town would go to traditional healers first for certain things and the medical doctors for other things. None of the traditional healers I studied with could say they hadn't gone themselves or sent one of their family members to a western doctor for certain things. They were tremendously open. They were always experimenting and always changing their system. It was more of a fluid system than the western system was. All plants had spirits and powers, but also the Earth, the Air, the Water and all of Nature.

Eliot: Tell me about the man you were closest to. What was his name?

Siri: His name was Tobae Agbaga Asou. He had a very interesting apprenticeship. He was taking a walk one day along a very rocky dirt road. An old man came up to him on a bike. It seemed amazing the old man could be riding a bike, there were so many rocks in the road. The man said, "Come back here tomorrow. I would like to show you something very important." He went back the next day and again the old man appeared on a bike, but this time on a nearby hill where they could hear drumming. It was wonderful drumming—some kind of ceremony. The man went with him to the top of the hill where the ceremony was, and people seemed to recognize him. They hugged him and were so happy to see him. He didn't recognize any of them. He was encouraged to stay there for a while, so he sat down. Then he felt a numbing in his body. He tried to get up but he couldn't move. He got very scared. The next thing he knew, he was going into the ground—deeper and deeper and deeper. He stayed there for nine Earth years!

Eliot: In what he called the Underworld?

Siri: He went to the very center of the earth. In that place were the most gifted teachers he had ever met. Those teachers taught him about herbs, about invoking spirits of herbs, and various aspects of healing. There were several dozen people who came to the Underworld at the same time to learn healing. The ones who could read and write took notes, and the ones who couldn't were tested every night to make sure they remembered. My friend was one of the group that had to be tested. I had interviewed many of his family members from the little village he lived in near Lomé and they talked about how he had disappeared. They thought he had been killed by some animal. He was gone for nine Earth years. Those nine years in the Underworld were like centuries. He said it was a different time sense there. The amount that he learned and the number of days were many more than nine years of regular Earth time. He learned lifetimes of information, particularly about the use of herbs. Then he came back and there was great rejoicing, and he became a healer. He was one of the most kind and bright and funny and empathic people I have met in my life.

He had tremendous humility. He also had a very strong sense of self—tremendous personal power. He had about thirty apprentices and about five hundred people came to his compound for healing every day. Just wall-to-wall people.

Eliot: How did he administer to all those people?

Siri: His apprentices did some of the work. At any time he had about thirty apprentices. He could look at people and sense what they needed. I stayed with him sometimes from two in the morning until two the next morning. He would be with people non-stop. He would tell his apprentices to prepare certain herbs for some people. For others, he would tell them where to pick certain herbs. Or he would give ceremonies to invoke spirit and the spirit would tell them what herbs to use and how to activate the spirits of these herbs. He treated everybody differently. With some people he would be very funny and they would be howling with laughter. With other people he wouldn't say anything; he would just listen. He might lecture and scream at his patients until they would cry. It would be a rapid succession of one group after another for at least twelve hours straight. He would get up every morning at about 3:30 and invoke different spirits of herbs and do certain chants. He would work on himself or purify himself for the work he had to do that day. Always the herbs were central to what he did.

Eliot: You mentioned once that many of his apprentices were well-respected healers in their own right.

Siri: Most of them had already achieved a high level of renown in their own villages before they went to him to study further about herbs. For him it wasn't simply the herb as we know it in the West, but it was the spirits associated with the herb. When you combine different herbs, then it brings different spirits than the spirits of the individual herbs.

Eliot: Would you recount the story of your extraordinary contact with him and his plant spirits?

Siri: I like to get up early in the morning and do yoga. In Togo, I did yoga from 3:30 until 6:00 every morning. I would do yoga and meditate and pray. No one had seen what I did. I had been going to this healer about three times a week to get interviews and to observe healing. Then after two or three months, he called me to him and said he felt very close to me and wanted to be friends, but he was in tremendous pain because he felt I had no idea who he really was. I couldn't understand who he was unless I could see and sense the spirits around him that were affecting him. Unless we know what powers are affecting a man, we can't really know who that man is. He would be happy to show me how to invoke plant spirits that would give me a vision of who he really was. So he asked me to come back in two weeks when he would have the proper herbs prepared. He also told me that he had been "coming to my apartment" since I arrived in the country. He was with me the two and a half hours I exercised in the mornings and he loved what I did. He told me in detail what he saw. He showed me some of the exercises I did—the Kundalini Yoga. He loved the kind of breathing I did. He loved the aroma of the flowers. He said they were very good for you. They were tuberoses. He said I had the wrong kind of incense and he would get me the correct incense. I was too limited in having just white candles; I needed seven different colors of candles.

Eliot:	In the flesh, he had never been to your apartment?
Siri:	That is correct. He had not been to my apartment in the flesh. Nor had anybody else from his group. No one had been to my apartment for my morning spiritual practice. No one had been there except for my wife. Actually, I wasn't surprised that he knew all of that. I felt closer to him. He knew so many details that I felt he had been to my house in the mornings.

He had the herbs waiting when I came back two weeks later. He could pick them out just perfectly with these strong massive hands, although they were dry and could crumble easily. The respect that he touched the herbs with really impressed me. It touched me in a way I hadn't been touched. Seeing his way of being with them communicated something important to me. He picked out three different herbs and told me to put all three leaves under each of the seven candles, to burn the incense he gave me while I did my usual two and a half hours of meditation and yoga practices. He told me some words to use at the end of my practices, to invoke the spirits in the plants, which would call upon his spirit. When I did that, my wife and I were together. We heard thunder and saw lightning in the room. We felt vibration and the roaring of a large animal. It seemed like a lion. In our minds' eyes, we saw crocodiles in the room. Both of us. I felt like he was in the room. I was seeing him as I hadn't seen him before. He was transparent. He let me go inside of his body. I felt pain in his chest from smoking a lot. I felt the body was ravaged by alcohol. But most of all, I felt the greatness of the person. I had never known a human could be so committed so continuously to serving other people. I never knew that a person could channel all the time, as he seemed to be. I also felt contradictions in him. Pain in his body. Dilemmas he was in. It was a very plausible picture of a full human being that I got.

When I went back to him, I told him what I saw and what I did. Then he confirmed that these animals were his protector animals. They were very important to him. Yes, his chest did hurt a lot. Nobody had told him he was smoking too much. Everybody was afraid to tell him what he was doing was wrong. He appreciated getting the feedback. The alcohol was terrible for his body in the quantities he had to consume, but the spirits who were linked to him wanted the alcohol. The only way they could get it was if he drank it. He would drink huge quantities every day. But whatever the reason for his drinking, he was a great man. He helped many people until his death last year.

Grandma Bertha Grove

I met Mrs. Bertha Grove at her home on the Southern Ute Reservation one icy autumn morning in 1991. As she opened the door to her modest house and greeted me with a warm smile, I immediately understood why people call her "Grandma." We went into her kitchen and unloaded the bags of groceries I had brought, and then she showed me into her parlor. She sat in an armchair beneath an enormous mounted buffalo head, and I installed myself in a sofa opposite her. Before she allowed me to switch on my tape recorder, she asked me to explain exactly what it was I wanted. I told her that I used the spirits of plants as medicine. I said that I thought it was important for people to know that plants have spirits that can heal, so I was writing a book about it, and I hoped that she would be willing to share some of her wisdom. She seemed satisfied, and nodding for me to begin recording, she chanted a long prayer in the Ute language. The interview that followed was both deep and broad, for Grandma Bertha spoke almost until midday. I transcribe here the parts that have to do with plant spirit medicine.

Bertha: That's what I have to do when somebody comes asking me something like that.... I have to say a prayer, have to ask the Grandfathers what you come looking for, what you want, because they know you, and they understand what it is that I have to tell you. I have to ask permission to say it; I don't just say it right off the bat.

It's the same way when we go gather the plants. There's different times and seasons to gather them. Some you can gather early in the morning, some at midday, some in the afternoon, and maybe the evening too. Some you gather at moonlight time, some in spring, some in summer, some in fall, some of the things we pick up in the winter, like cedar. We don't just go over there and start choppin' or pickin'. When we go, we take tobacco or whatever gift that I'm going to give to them.

Supposing you're the cedar. It's just like I'm asking you a favor, asking for your help, asking for some of your clothing or your limbs. We tell you why we're going to use it, what we're going to do for people. When I say that and get the OK, then I give my gift. I usually tie a scarf. Whenever I see a sale, I usually buy some scarves; that way I have some all the time, and I keep them and some tobacco in my car, because you never know what plants I'm going to find.

Once you got your permission, you just take what you need. Never be greedy—that's one of the rules. If you need some, get what you need, and if you have to get some for people, get that too, but you have to ask that you're going to take more than you're going to use, because you are going to give some to the people. And that's the way we do it. I don't know, is that the way you do things?

Eliot: Yes, yes.

Bertha: Supposing you're using the leaves or the branches or the stems…. You make a tea or a poultice, and then what do you do with it after?

Eliot: I find that the main thing is to get the permission of the spirit that is going to help me help others. If I can make that relationship with the spirit of the plant, I don't need the leaf or the root or whatever. Sometimes I can ask the spirit of the plant to come through my hands….

Bertha: But you don't actually use the plant to make a tea?

Eliot: One of my main helpers is like a messenger, so I make a tincture of the messenger and I ask the messenger to bring the spirit of whatever plant that person needs. So instead of having dozens of plants that I have to take with me, I just have pills made out of the messenger plant.

Bertha: Like you say, everything has a spirit. The plants and trees and rocks are people, too. It's good the way you do things. I tell people it's good that they learn different ways of doing things. They can teach others, and I teach my way and it's all to help heal people.

Eliot:	How do you find out how a certain plant can help?
Bertha:	Mostly it's your guardian spirit, your inner self that tells you. You and I, we really don't know anything. It's the spirits that work through us; we're just the instrument these things work through. I have to ask the Creator to help me, and whatever way He tells me to do it, that's the way I'll move around. It might not be the same for different persons. Each person has their own body, mind and spirit, and so the treatment is individual. It would be different for another person with the same ailment. It's the same when you talk to people; you have to treat them individually.
Eliot:	Do you ever ask the spirits of the plants?
Bertha:	That's what I'm asking for when I'm out there gathering the plant. I'm talking to the spirit of that plant. Have you seen them spirits?
Eliot:	Yeah. Do the plants tell you how to use them?
Bertha:	Uh huh, they tell you. The spirit that you're talking about is universally in everything. That's why you have to have respect for animals and birds and plants. You know, even Mother Earth has got a lot of power in her. That's what I try to tell people: walk sacredly on Mother Earth. Mother Earth knows you—where you've been, where you're coming from. The spirits of everything are everywhere, surrounding us. You're watched by a thousand eyes every day, every move you make. So you ask permission when you're out there. You ask the Creator and you talk to Mother Earth and you talk to the Four Directions because you're using all of it. That plant did not come by itself. It came by Mother Earth. The Sun came up and warmed it. The blessing is in there. The Rain fell on it to make it grow, so you thank the Thunder Beings and the Cloud People for letting this plant grow. You thank the wind that blew, and you ask the Four Grandfathers and Grandmothers in the Four Directions for permission. This plant has spirit, and it didn't get spirit by itself. The Creator is the one who put it there. Anybody can use it; all you have to do is ask for help. You don' have to carry medicine bags around; just use what is in front of you. It's there to help people. It's got power: sticks, rocks,

Mother Earth, even the wind has power. You can help people like that.

Like you said, it can come through your hand. Your hand is the most powerful thing you have. It's used to help people, to bless people, so you can't hit anybody with it, right? But that's good, you use your hands that way.

Like I say, there's many ways of helping people: through the plants, the water…you can use anything in this world. Like the hair of that Grandfather. [She points to the buffalo head on the wall above her.] One old Taos man gave me that for people who are going out of their mind. He said, "Keep it, one day you might use it." So different people have taught me, different tribes, you know.

Eliot: Could you talk a little more about how you learned?

Bertha: Oh, well…I grew up with my grandfather and he was a Medicine Man, one of the Ute. When a couple had more children than they could take care of in the old days, one was given to the grandparents or to the uncle or aunt. I was given to my grandparents, and they raised me. He was a Medicine Man and I grew up in that atmosphere. I grew up in a teepee, one of the last teepees on the reservation, so I know how to live in a teepee, how you're supposed to be in there, and how you're supposed to be with a Medicine Man. What I didn't understand until I was older was that to each of us—there were five that he had given the gift to—there was going to come a time when we would use it. I started dreaming, you know….

Eliot: How old were you?

Bertha: When it first began I was still in my teens. This thing would talk to me and I'd get scared. They told me, "The Creator chose you to do His work." And I made a prayer and I said, "No, I'm too young. I can't do this work." So it kind of went away. Then I had kids; I had my children when I was real young.

Eliot: You prayed that this gift be taken away?

Bertha: Yeah, I was scared of it. So in my twenties, it came back again. I said, "I got kids to raise; I got no time for this. Wait till my hair turns gray." It said, "OK." But in the meantime, people are coming to me telling me a lot of things I should know...elderly people from different tribes. I'm not out there seeking for it, they're coming to me, and I'm learning, I'm seeing things in a gradual sort of way.

Well, in my early thirties, my hair turned gray. "You said 'wait till my hair turns gray', and it's gray now!" ...that's what that spirit told me. I said, "Wait a while." Then I got sick. I got asthma, I got crippled up with arthritis, couldn't walk, couldn't work any more. My husband said, "Maybe you ought to listen to what they tell you."

Then I started dreaming of Sun Dance. I'd never seen women sundance, but I'd helped my husband and my boys into the Sun Dance ceremony, 'cause my grandfather that raised me was a Sun Dance chief. I'd been helping him since I was a little girl. They made me do things that was teaching me, I guess. I thought I was being treated mean...the hardships I had in my childhood....

I used to herd sheep when I was little, you know. Way out there in the hills, all by myself, with just my dog and the sheep. You know, you sit out there in the hills and you're wondering about everything. That was part of the stuff that I was supposed to learn...observing nature, the plants. I was talking to them because I had nobody else to talk to. I'd see them rocks, pick them up, talk to them, put them back. They were my playmates. Flowers, rocks and brush and whatever were my playmates. I didn't realize I was being taught.

I started Sun Dancing. One day I had a dream that said, "Now's the time." I'd worked for the BIA [Bureau of Indian Affairs] for so long, I said "I can't just up and quit." But the dream told me I had to quit now, take them white man's shoes off, put on moccasins. For four years I wore those moccasins through spring and fall, summer and winter, because the spirit told me I could never put no shoes on. Then I went Sun Dancing, and that's where my physical body began to come back into shape again. I couldn't get up by myself, but my husband came over early to the arbor where we were dancing, and I was already up, and he said, "How did you get up?" "I got up," I said.

You know that asthma went away. I always tell people I'm a testament to what plants can do for you, what spirits can do for you, what faith can do for you. At my age—I'm almost seventy—I can move faster than most younger ones. I can get up, walk a long ways, take care of our house, cook for us, which I'm grateful for.

I was trained for who and what I was, and I knew why those old people had been showing me. It all came together little by little. One old man, he's from the Northern Utes, he helped me a lot, made me understand about the spirits. And I have another from up there, he taught me a lot about the spirits, the Grandfathers, the Grandmothers, about the sweat lodges. Some of it I learned through Sun Dancing and through my vision quests.

The way I see it, everything is good; the Creator said He made everything good, and it's still the same way. It is just man that thinks, "That plant is no good; that animal is no good." There is a reason for Him creating it. There is a reason for snakes, for flies. We say spray the heck out of them, but I found out if you talk to them they won't bother you any more.

These spirits are real. If you believe in them, they'll help you. That is what those medical doctors don't understand. They could do a lot of things if they could just believe in this Creation, in the spirits. Maybe there are a few who know that, but very few. Even in our own clinic they think we're crazy if we talk about that. Lot of people think you're crazy if you do things like that. I guess you come up against that....

Eliot:	I usually don't tell people that the spirits are helping. Maybe they wouldn't be there if they knew.
Bertha:	It doesn't bother me what people think, because I've had my experiences. I was told, "Never mind if people laugh at you, call you names. Don't worry about that. You do My work for me. I'm the one you'd better be scared of; I'm the one that's making you do this work, helping you." So that's what I do—is follow the Creator. If somebody asks me for help, I pray about it first. If I'm supposed to help, I will. If I'm not, then I'll get somebody else.

Eliot: Your dreams, are they nighttime dreams or daytime dreams?

Bertha: Whenever I sleep. If they're nighttime dreams, then I wake up (afterwards). Sometimes they're daytime dreams. You think you're dreaming, but you're not. If it's quiet, I can meditate or I'm doing something, but I'm like dreaming, seeing things. Sometimes I can close my eyes and talk real quiet and I can see. If I go to a ceremony, I can talk to Grandfather Fire; I can talk to the Grandfathers and they'll show me. It's like a TV there.

These things don't lie, you know. People can lie, but the Creation can't lie. So if a plant spirit is talking to you and you're absorbing it, then you do what it tells you to do. You don't go beyond, adding little fringes to it, or something like that. Maybe someone expects you to do more, but it's like, "This is what I'm supposed to do, and that's it." That's all.

Eliot: Could you talk about when you healed somebody using a plant?

Bertha: OK...Let's see, there are so many.... OK, I'm going to leave some part out, just tell you other parts....

One time there was this family in Taos, and this lady's uncle was having a hard time, because somebody burnt down his house and his trading post. Well, about two, three years before we'd been down there, and she called me "Mother," you know. She took me to see her uncle at his trading post; we didn't know him then. She introduced us, and he gave me a shawl out of his store, a red and blue shawl for one of the ceremonies that we have. There's stories behind that, too. He gave my husband a gourd, my friend a feather, different stuff like that. So we thanked him.

So years later, he's having a problem and they told us to come down there and do a ceremony for him. So my husband and I took off. I'm driving over Tres Piedras, up that big mountain. When I got way on top, all of a sudden something tells me, "Turn around!" So, quick, I turned around and stopped. There's this aspen tree and I told my husband, "I'm supposed to get something here." He said, "OK." That's one thing about him, he never questions. So we got out, and I told him, "We need four branches, four twigs from the top of the tree."

Eliot: The tree told you that?

Bertha: Yes. See, I don't know why I'm doing this; I'm just doing what the tree is telling me. So my husband is hanging up there, and the grandchildren are laughing: "Hey, Grandpa is like a monkey!" So he pulls the branches over to me and I cut them off and do my prayers. I put water on the towel I carry with me, and I wrap it away. I don't know what I'm going to do with it.

So we get down there into Taos and they're having the ceremony, and the branches are still in the van. Then, after midnight, "Hey, that plant is talking again!" So I tell my husband, "Go get that plant for me," and he went and got it. I'm just doing what the branches are telling me, so I go up to these people I don't know and I say, "You Taos people use aspen in your ceremonies, your feasts, your kivas, and at this time, I'm going to ask you to use these aspen branches to help that person standing over there. Use this; bless him with it." They said, "Alright," and got everything situated.

At that time I didn't know that man. I didn't know that he was the uncle of the person we were doing the ceremony for. I didn't know that this man didn't like his nephew, and that he did him wrong. All I knew was the plant is telling me to give it to that man. And he gets up there, and he starts to pray. He's talking in his own language, but the ladies told me the next morning, they said: "How did you know? How did you know he was the one who burned down his house and store?" I said: "I didn't know. I was just doing what the plant was telling me to do." They told me that in his prayer he was confessing, that he was sorry that he had hurt him like that.

He told me the next morning, "When I was touched by that branch, it was so powerful...the energy just come and shook me and I wanted to scream or howl, but I held myself. I could feel that force. It made me tremble like a lightning strike or something."

I told the man who was blessing him, "You keep it, and sometime before three days are over you take it back up on that mountain where nobody goes around, and you thank it for the blessing you got."

The next morning that uncle was trying to make him give the branches to him, saying, "I'll put it in the kiva; it's really powerful." But I told him, "It's not going to do anything unless the spirit is with it. It won't do anything unless you're doing what it tells you to do. The plant said it came through here, and now it's got to go up there, up in the mountains, back where it belongs."

And that man who the ceremony was for, he got alright—built another store, he became the War Chief, became Governor, he's doing alright, see?

That's what that plant can do for you: make a way for you like that. You just have to keep your mind, your heart, your spirit open to the creation so you can hear these things.

So that was one time that we helped with aspen leaves. Sometimes I use sage.

Eliot:	Do you have a good sage story?
Bertha:	Lots of things I do, I don't remember them. You're not supposed to, I guess; you just do it…. Let's see, a sage story…. We were on our way to Utah one time, and I said, "Stop!" I told my husband, "Over there; pick four of them, just four." So he did.
Eliot:	This is sage?
Bertha:	Yes, four of those little sages. We took that sage—where we were going was to another ceremony this lady was having for herself.
Eliot:	Was she ill?
Bertha:	She was ill; she was diabetic. Her legs were swelling up so that she couldn't walk. So I told them: "Use that sage on her." So, by morning her leg was normal size. She got up and walked out. You just rub it; you kind of press it on her.
	There's a lot of ways to help people, lots of ways. Sometimes we put it on a patient and blow into it. Peppermint is good that way too.
Eliot:	How do you mean, blow into it?

Bertha: What I do is I dip it in running water four times, and ask the Creation, Four Directions and Mother Earth. Before you put it in the water, ask Grandmother Water for help. You're asking everything to support that Grandmother. That's a Grandmother too, that female sage. That one is real pretty. You just put it on [the patient's skin] and blow into it.

Sometimes when I use the sage like that, I take out whatever is in there: the pain. You'd be amazed what you'd find, some of the things that people do to each other. Maybe you'd know, maybe you don't. They call it witchcraft. You can take that out, too.

See, the Creation and the Four Directions, they're real powerful and they're supporting that sage, and you're supporting it too, with your breath, because you are a spirit, too. All spirits have to work together—the spirit of the plants and everything. Sometimes you need support, and even that plant needs the support of the Mother Earth where it came from. So you learn.... You're learning. Maybe you have learned more than me.

But like I say, I'm not just a plant [healer], I'm the whole thing, the whole Creation.

The Grandfather, he's the one you have to talk to, the one you have to ask, because he's the Creator, and you always have to ask his permission...to use the spirit of this plant here. Then you gotta thank the spirit of the plant, then you gotta thank the Creator and Mother Earth where it comes from. You gotta learn to be appreciative of things.

Do you see them plant spirits around you?

Eliot: When I close my eyes and relax. Usually I use drumming to help me; then I can see the spirits.

Bertha: Yeah, that's what we do in our ceremonies. Someone is drumming. That's good, you know.

Once you begin to know the spirits, you begin to put things in their place, as time comes along....

We use the sage for smudging a lot, for blessing. It helps clean out the things from around you that block your spirit. Do you do anything besides talking to the spirits when you're helping people? Do you go through some formalities?

Eliot:	Not usually. When you're dealing with white people in the city, you start to do those things and....
Bertha:	You can't do anything the way they understand.
Eliot:	So the other things I keep to myself.
Bertha:	That's good. I'm glad you do that. I got to do that, too, with my white people. [Laughs] I got to learn to do it like that when I work with white people.
Eliot:	Well, people who come to you are open-minded.
Bertha:	Yeah, a lot of times I'll give them a brief explanation of why I'm using this, why I'm doing this. That way they can have a little bit of understanding of it. I'm glad you're working in that way. That's a new thing. See, I learned from you. I'm going to put that into practice! We ask the spirit, but asking the plant to do the work [of collecting and delivering the medicine], hey, that takes a lot off me! [laughs] Make it work, make the plant work, instead of me doing it! Anyway, I'm glad to meet you. I hope I told you what you wanted to know.
Eliot:	This has been wonderful!
Bertha:	Like I say, the plants was human one time and they gave their life, their spirits, because we're asking them for help. It's just like the food we eat. It was alive, one time it was moving around, and it gave up. That's why I tell them when you go hunting, you have to talk to the spirit of the wild animals, thank them, because they gave their lives. Even that fire: that tree was a living thing, was growing. So when you build a fire, think about it. It gave its life so you could have heat. Even the coal, gas, butane, came out of Mother Earth; it's part of her. Even the water you drink. People don't look at it like that. That's why people contaminate it. They don't understand. The Water of Life, that's what the Indians call it. We have great respect for it. I learned from experience, so I go back and say thank you. The Water of Life, some of it comes from within the Mother Earth, but, hey, government is taking it all away from us. They're even in the underground waters now. My Grandfather told me, "Way down the line, they're gonna be fighting over water. You keep your Indian way of life. Maybe you can save some of your people

that way, when the time comes. I'm not going to be around, but these ways might help you save yourself and some of your people when the time comes."

A lot of people wonder why I talk to people like you. They say I'm giving away knowledge of Indian people. But there's lots of Indian people that's trying to share our beliefs with people of other cultures so that you can understand me and I can understand you. If we don't include the spiritual part, then we can't understand each other.

You have your culture. They used plants, too—way back. In European countries, they had the knowledge of the plants. So I tell people, "You have it, too, this isn't just my secret or Indians' secret. You have a right to know, because you had it, too. It's just that somewhere along the line it got lost. You just need to recapture it, and when you do, we'll get along."

Eliot: It's so important to start learning from Mother Earth again.

Bertha: Uh huh, I learned a long time ago about owning things. Pretty soon they own you. You gotta make payments. So a lot of people are going back to a simple way of living. Because really, we make it hard for ourselves. That's what one old man told me, "There's nothing to life." He said, "Sun comes up, we get up, do our prayers, and we eat breakfast. Through the day we do what we have to do—go visit people or go work. Then evening comes, sun goes down, we come back home, eat again, talk...whatever we done all through the day, we talk about it. Then we go to bed, make our prayers again, sleep. Then the sun comes up, we do it again, go through life. We make it hard for our own self 'cause we put in all these worries. We make our own problems. But it's really simple. You just live. Enjoy yourself." That's what he told me.

He was right. I live that way now. I'm not in a hurry. I don't rush around. Frustration, hate, bitterness will take a physical toll on you. That's what's gonna make you sick. Cancer, tumors, diabetes is caused by all these things you put on your own self. Heart trouble, stroke...hate and bitterness causes strain on your heart.

Don't do it. It doesn't matter what anybody says—that's their problem. Don't carry it.

Now I just say, "Grandfather, take care of it, whatever's not right."

Us Indians don't have no devil or hell. It isn't that way. It's just our thoughts that make it that way. The way I'm telling you is the way I was taught, the way I was shown. I could sit back here and make up lies, stories about the plants, the miracles I've done. But it wasn't that way. You would believe me, 'cause I'm an elder, but I can't do it that way. I have to tell the truth the way I've experienced it. If I lie to you I have to answer to that Person up there. That's one I'm very respectful of, very fearful of what that would do. If you lie, you have to live with it. In time it's going to affect your mind and your body, so why lie? So you be yourself, that's what I tell people. That's what I tell you.

I hope I have been of help to you, a little bit anyway. I've done something in the name of the Creation, the Grandfathers and the plants...on their behalf.

You have gone a long way into the plant things. Even herbalists don't go that far. They just use it like giving you an aspirin. They give you a capsule, but they really haven't gone to that spirit. But you have. You have that messenger.... That's something for me to think about. I have learned something from you, and I appreciate it. As time goes on, I'll think about it, and say, "That's what he was talking about."

That's about all I could say to you. I want to thank you for coming. In talking to you, I help myself. It's not very often I come across people who have the power and the energy to do this kind of work with the spirits.

Eliot: I think it's that most people don't have the interest.

Bertha: Maybe that's why. You have that knowledge; you'll go on with this. "Don't get too proud," I tell people. "Don't be getting in front of people. Stay back. Be humble."

Epilogue

When I finished writing this book, I accompanied Don Guadalupe González Ríos on his first trip outside Mexico. He performed startling healings and I served as translator during his tour of the Western United States. One evening we found ourselves traveling in a car in the company of Grandma Bertha Grove and a few friends. I had not seen Grandma Bertha in some time, and she was questioning me about my work with the Huichol shaman. I told her he was guiding me on a six-year training in the medicine of a sacred tree that grows on a remote mountain peak.

"What do they call that tree?" Grandma asked.

"In Don Lupe's language they call it 'kieri,'" I said. "In English, it means 'the wind tree.'"

"The wind tree!" exclaimed Grandma Bertha. "You say it grows on a mountain top? What does it look like?"

"The one I work with isn't a tree, really. It's a small shrub."

"You mean it hasn't grown up to be a tree yet?"

"No, it's fully grown," I said, "but it's just a little shrub."

"I thought you said it was a tree."

"Well, it could be a tree. I guess it could be most any kind of plant. When a certain spirit comes to live inside a plant, that plant becomes the wind tree. It doesn't matter what species it is."

"When I was younger," Grandma said, "there was an old man who used to teach me. He was from the Northern Utes. He's not alive anymore. Anyway, when there was something important I wanted to know, I'd go see him. He didn't have no telephone, he couldn't read or write, but he knew when I was coming. He would be there waiting for me.

"So this one time I had the same dream four nights in a row. I figured it was important, so I decided to go see this old man to ask him about it. In the dream, I went to a house out in the country. When I got inside, there were four old women in there. They danced and did ceremony and gave me this stick of wood about a foot and half long. They said I was supposed to have it.

"When I got to the old man's house, he was waiting for me just like he always was. We sat down and talked about my family, about this and that. You know how it is with the old people—you have to be patient; you have to be respectful. I never said nothing about why I was there. So after about three hours, he says, 'That stick they gave you in your dreams—you're supposed to have it, you're supposed to heal people with it. It comes form a very powerful tree that grows way high on the top of a certain mountain. They call it the lightning tree. You wait here; I'm going to get that stick for you.' I waited. Three days later, he came back with a stick from the lightning tree. This was years ago. I still have that stick. I hardly ever take it out. Time hasn't come yet, I guess."

"It's interesting he called it the lightning tree," I said, "because lightning has a lot to do with the wind tree, too. Don Lupe tells the story that the wind tree was originally a little baby boy. He was a real nuisance because he cried all the time. His parents couldn't get any sleep, they couldn't get their work done because he just cried and cried. One night they got so fed up they took him out on the patio and threw a blanket over his head and left him there. During the night Trickster came and led him off into the mountains. Eventually, the boy turned himself into a tree that grows on a high cliff—the wind tree.

"The next day the father came back from working in the fields and checked on his son, but, of course, he was gone. The mother and father looked everywhere for their boy, but all they found was a miniature set of deer antlers next to a shrub on a high cliff.

"Some wise shamans were called in. They spent the night chanting by the shrub. Around one or two in the morning, the child appeared to them. His parents didn't care for him, he said, so he had gone off to the mountains with his friend Trickster and become a tree. But he said that the shamans should tell his parents that in five days he would return to visit them.

"Five days later, there was an incredible storm with powerful winds and rays of lightning streaking across the sky. The parents were disappointed not to see their son. Once more the shamans were summoned and spoke to the boy. He explained that he had visited his parents in the form of lightning and wind. They would never see him again in human form.

"Later on in the story, the boy becomes an old man who appears on the mountain top and declares that he will grant the gift of healing or any other knowledge. He takes the form of a lightning bolt and rises into the sky. Then he becomes an eagle and flies away."

"What a bizarre story!" said my friend Roxanne. "What do you make of it, Eliot?"

"I haven't checked this out with the master here," I said, "but I think it's an allegory of the shaman's apprenticeship."

"How is that?"

"All the different characters are parts of the apprentice, parts of me. Mother and Father trying to do their chores represent the normal work-a-day me. The baby represents the undeveloped potential of my soul that cries out for attention. But the square part of me can't understand the crying of my soul, doesn't like it, throws a blanket over it. Might as well be a wet blanket. My neglected soul gets disenchanted, turns away from normal human life, and gets led into the wilderness by Trickster. In the wilderness my soul begins to rediscover its power— symbolized by lightning and wind. I try to show this to Mom and Dad, but they don't get it, so eventually my soul realizes it's not about getting approval, it's about becoming a fountain of blessing for the community. This is gaining maturity, thus the baby boy becomes a wise old man.

"There is more, but we can talk about it some other time. What I'm wondering is: could the wind tree and the lightning tree be the same thing?"

Until now, Don Lupe had been quietly looking out the window of the speeding car. I turned to him and recounted in Spanish Grandma Bertha's story about the lightning tree. "Is this really the wind tree?" I asked.

"Tell her to bring me the stick next time we meet," Don Lupe said. "If it makes my hand tremble when I hold it, it is the wind tree. If not, it isn't."

His answer raised tantalizing questions in my mind. Until now the wind tree had seemed to be the esoteric knowledge of a small tribe in Mexico, but perhaps Grandma Bertha had been introduced to it in a dream as I had been. Her mentor obviously had known about it. If the Utes know the wind tree, could it not be possible that other North American tribes do too? And if that is the case, might not the incredible power of wind tree be known and used by traditional peoples in other parts of the world as well?

A few days later, Don Lupe announced his plans to retire in two years, leaving the guidance of the other wind tree apprentices in my hands. If I am to be ready to take on the job, the next two years will be the most intense, the most interesting of my life! The past thirty years have been an introduction, I realized, and the book on plant spirit medicine has not yet been written.

Suggestions for Further Reading

My approach to plant spirit medicine is practical rather than scholarly, so this is not a definitive bibliography but instead a list of a few books I find helpful.

As far as I know, there is virtually nothing in print on the use of plant spirits for healing, but if you read Spanish you would probably enjoy the anecdotes about Mexican herbalists in *Acerca de Plantas y de Curanderos* by Bernardo Baytelman, Instituto Nacional de Antropologloia e Historia, Mexico D.F. 1993.

The subject of shamanism has recently produced a huge volume of literature whose quality varies enormously. *Shamanic Voices* (Dutton, 1979) by Joan Halifax is one of my favorites, and I highly recommend the magazine *Shaman's Drum*, P. O. Box 430, Willits, CA 95490. Sandra Ingermann's book, entitled *Soul Retrieval* (Harper San Francisco 1991), is excellent for more information on this particular technique of shamanistic healing.

If you were intrigued by Don Enrique Salmon's description of Native American paths of knowledge, you would enjoy *Trail to Heaven*, a lively account of Beaver Indian epistemology by anthropologist Robin Ridington (University of Iowa Press, 1988).

For more background on classical Chinese medical theory, I recommend three books by my teacher, Professor J. R. Worsley: *Is Acupuncture for You?*, *Talking About Acupuncture*, and *Traditional Acupuncture Volume II: Traditional Diagnosis*. All three are available from the Worsley Institute of Classical Acupuncture, 6175 NW 153 St., Suite 324, Miami Lakes, Florida 33104.

If you are planning to do field work with wild plants and need help identifying species, the *Peterson Field Guides* (Boston: Houghton Mifflin) are the best for amateurs.

Turbulent Mirror by Briggs & Peat (Harper & Row, New York, 1989) is an account of the new scientific field of chaos theory. If you enjoy speculating about the common ground of modern science and ancient healing practices, this book will stimulate you.

Where to Go From Here

If you are interested in short courses or professional trainings in plant spirit medicine, if you would like a referral to a practitioner in your area, or for more information regarding pilgrimages to places of power, please write:

Eliot Cowan
775 E. Blithedale, #203
Mill Valley, CA 94941

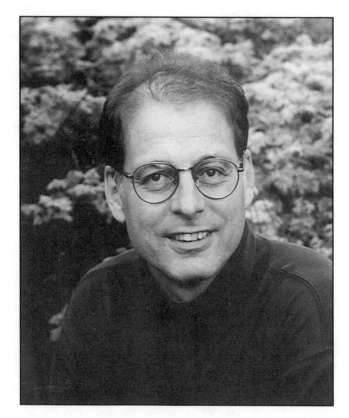

Eliot Cowan

Biography

Eliot Cowan was born in 1946 and was raised in Chicago, Winnipeg and San Francisco. He graduated in anthropology from Pomona College and did post-graduate studies in ethnographic documentary filmmaking at UCLA.

Eliot began to study and practice herbalism in 1969, and set it aside after a few years to study acupuncture. He received his Licentiate, Bachelor and Master of Acupuncture degrees from J. R. Worsley at the College of Traditional Acupuncture, Leamington Spa, England, and served on the faculty of that institution in 1979-80.

In the early 1980s, Eliot once again turned his attention to herbal healing. This time he was instructed directly by the spirits of the herbs. Together with his plant mentors, Cowan rediscovered the ancient shamanic practice of plant spirit medicine.

Currently Eliot Cowan is the apprentice and designated successor of Don Guadalupe González Ríos, an elder Huichol Indian shaman and plant spirit healer. Mr. Cowan lives with his family in Mexico and devotes his time to plant spirit medicine teaching and practice in Mexico, the United States and abroad.

CALLING THE CIRCLE

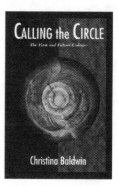

The First and Future Culture

BY CHRISTINA BALDWIN

The Circle has been used as a spiritual and social form since the first campfires. People gather into circles to call on spirit, to celebrate, to hold council, to create community, to govern by consensus, to make cooperative decisions and take action.

In her definitive new work, activist author Christina Baldwin introduces a structure for calling the circle and exploring its potential to empower us in our ordinary lives.

"The circle is an ancient form whose time has come again, and Baldwin is a brilliant spokesperson for this reclamation."

> Vicki Noble
> Author of Shakti Woman

"A reminder of the basic protocols and commitments necessary for enriching collective work and making significant contributions in teams, families and growth circles."

> Angeles Arrian, Ph.D.
> Author of The Four-Fold Way

"This is a worthy and practical book for these times which demand a spiritual reawakening."

> Mathew Fox
> Author of The Reinvention of Work

ISBN 0-932310-8-1
Tradepaper, 252 pages
Retail $14.95

Swan•Raven & Co.
P. O. Box 726
Newberg, OR 97132
800-366-0264

Ritual

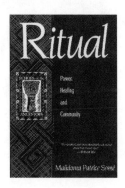

Power, Healing
and Community

BY MALIDOMA SOMÉ

Ritual describes the kinds of expected interactions between the ancestral spiritual world and this one, the uses and dangers of traditional ritual practice, and how it is performed.

Malidoma Somé, spokesman for the Dagara Ancestors, lives in three worlds: the world of his village, the world of the Ancestors and the modern Western world. Holder of two Ph.D.'s, he considers his traditional initiation into ancestral knowledge his true education. Told by the elder of his village that the Ancestors wanted him to go the the West, he immersed himself in Western culture. Malidoma now acts as a bridge between these three worlds, bringing the teachings of the Ancestors to echo within our own souls.

> *"This is the greatest and most detailed book about ritual that I have read.... At a time when the West needs to relearn ritual for its own healing, this book is valuable, lively and sound."*
>
> —Robert Bly
> *Author of* Iron John

ISBN 0-9632310-3-0
Tradepaper, 150 pages
Retail $12.95

Swan•Raven & Co.
P. O. Box 726
Newberg, OR 97132
800-366-0264

When Sleeping Beauty Wakes Up

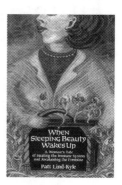

A Woman's Tale of Healing the Immune System and Awakening the Feminine

BY PATT LIND-KYLE

When Sleeping Beauty Wakes Up is the story of a near-death journey of emotional healing and spiritual awakening through a long illness with Chronic Fatigue Syndrome. By going through a life and death process, the author uncovered a new path to a woman's feminine strength and discovered a simple healing system. Her research with professional women presents the loss of true feminine experience in our culture and how women can return to an inward presence to have stronger self-esteem, self-image and knowledge of the transforming feminine.

> *"Hers is not only a literal story of her battle with a 'woman's disease,' but also a metaphorical telling about the condition of many American women today, whose efforts toward healing are really attempts to reclaim their power in a subtly, but insidiously, male-dominated culture."*
>
> —*Laurie Wimmer*
> *Executive Director*
> *Oregon Commission on Women*

ISBN 0-9632310-1-4
Tradepaper, 256 pages
Retail $14.95

Swan•Raven & Co.
P. O. Box 726
Newberg, OR 97132
800-366-0264

Human Robots & Holy Mechanics

Reclaiming Our Souls in a Machine World

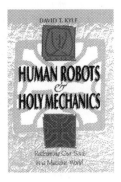

BY DAVID T. KYLE

We are trapped in a mechanized consumer-driven society. The corporation-economy creates a Machine culture in which all of us are oilers of our spiritual impoverishment. We have been cut off from the Sacred—the connection with an Otherworld of spiritual reality that comes to us through Nature. Indigenous people and our archaic ancestors hold fundamental beliefs and ways of relating to the physical and non-physical world that we've lost in our society of the Machine. By initiating elder-leaders, establishing epiphanal communities, fasting from the media and mapping the topography of our inner experience, we begin to reclaim from the Machine the Sacred, and conceive a different future for ourselves, our children and our planet.

"This heartfelt book brings important insights, drawn from years of experience, to challenges we will all have to face if we are to move beyond today's corporate culture to a genuinely positive future."

—*Robert Gilman*
Publisher, In-Context Magazine

ISBN 0-9632310-0-6
Tradepaper, 300 pages
Retail $14.95

Swan•Raven & Co.
P. O. Box 726
Newberg, OR 97132

The Swan and the Raven traditionally carry the Sacred Message between the Otherworld and our world. Swan•Raven & Company publishes books whose themes explore this Sacred Message.

If you would like to receive our latest catalog and be placed on our mailing list, please send the enclosed card.

Name _____ Date_____

Address_____

City _____ State_____ Zip _____

Country _____

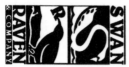

Swan•Raven & Co.
P.O. Box 726
Newberg, Oregon 97132

DATE DUE

APR 7 '98	AP 25		
JUN 14 '98			
JUN 14 '98	2/28/11		
ILL			
KH			
5/4/00			
JUN 1 3 2000			
ILL			
Kimball			
11/26/00			
AP 3 0			
5/12/01			
OCT 2 3 2001			
APR 2 5 2002			
NO 01 '02			